ARE YOU SUFFERING FROM
A REPETITIVE MOTION DISORDER?

THIS BOOK WILL SHOW YOU HOW TO:

- RECOGNIZE the early symptoms so that you can get prompt treatment.

- FIND the best medical specialists in the field.

- ASK the right questions about diagnostic tests, conservative therapies, and surgery.

- TAKE STEPS to make your work environment safer and to prevent recurrence of your injury.

- ENLIST the aid of government agencies that regulate safety in the workplace.

- AND MUCH MORE!

With the help of this clear, comprehensive, and reassuring guide, you can put an end to your pain—now and forever!

RELIEF FROM CARPAL TUNNEL SYNDROME
and Other Repetitive Motion Disorders

THE DELL MEDICAL LIBRARY

Relief from
CARPAL TUNNEL SYNDROME
and Other Repetitive
Motion Disorders

Norra Tannenhaus

Foreword by Eric Carlson, M.D.

A LYNN SONBERG BOOK

Published by
Dell Publishing
a division of
Bantam Doubleday Dell Publishing Group, Inc.
666 Fifth Avenue
New York, New York 10103

Medical research about carpal tunnel syndrome and other repetitive motion disorders is ongoing and subject to interpretation. Although every effort has been made to include the most up-to-date and accurate information in this book, there can be no guarantee that what we know about these subjects today won't change with time. The reader should bear in mind that this book is not for the purpose of self-diagnosis or self-treatment and should consult appropriate medical professionals regarding all problems related to their health.

ISBN: 0-440-20979-X

Printed by arrangement with Lynn Sonberg Book Services, 166 East 56 Street, New York, New York 10022

Printed in the United States of America

Published simultaneously in Canada

October 1991

10 9 8 7 6 5 4 3 2 1

OPM

CONTENTS

A Note to the Reader: This book contains quotes from, and case histories of, people who have carpal tunnel syndrome and similar disorders. The names of these people have been changed to protect their privacy.

FOREWORD

Eric Carlson, M.D.

Not too long ago people questioned the causes of carpal tunnel syndrome, despite compelling evidence that the condition was related to repetitive motion on the job. But as the 1990s progress and the incidence of carpal tunnel syndrome (CTS) continues to rise, its origins have become increasingly clear. Each year workers lose countless days from work—indeed a few unfortunates lose their jobs altogether—and industry loses millions of dollars in productivity, medical costs, and workers' compensation claims, all because of CTS. Companies also incur expenses through making changes in the workplace to reduce the risk of CTS, or through government-imposed sanctions if they do not.

As you'll learn in this book, CTS is fairly simple for an experienced physician to diagnose and treat. In most cases its symptoms are characteristic and treatment is clear-cut; splints and various kinds of medication, followed by surgery if those do not work. And although some rare horror stories may make the evening news, the vast majority of people with CTS do well after they are treated.

Unfortunately this does not address the real question, which is how can ordinary people protect themselves from the pain, expense, and inconvenience of CTS? As this book tells you, the answer lies in assessing your job, your workplace, and the other activities you regularly perform in order to identify and if possible eliminate the actions that may lead to CTS or one of its related disorders, which are also discussed in this book. Some things you can do on your own; others require the cooperation of your fellow workers or perhaps even the managers of your company. It also requires companies to assume their fair share of responsibility to provide their employees with a workplace that eliminates risk as much as possible. This may sound like a tall order, but as you will see, it's far less costly for industry to make changes before problems occur than it is to deal with the consequences later.

Progress is a mixed blessing. It has permitted enormous increases in productivity, and sometimes in creativity as well, and has liberated many workers from jobs that might otherwise be far more tedious or even hazardous. On the other hand it has also led to a rise in CTS and similar problems, for reasons described in the book. Labor and management must work together to find ways of protecting the work force. The good news is that many industries have voluntarily made changes to diminish these risks, and government agencies are more vigilant than ever in assuring workers' rights to a safe job site. The 1990s are opening with an epidemic of CTS, but very possibly they will close with American workers being safer than they ever were before.

INTRODUCTION

For Shelly it began in October 1988. Then a reporter for a newspaper, she began feeling pain from her hand all the way up her arm. A doctor diagnosed it as stress.

A few months later Shelly moved to another state where, as a reporter for a large urban newspaper, she began a grueling assignment, requiring a lot of time and legwork. She wrote at a computer whose keyboard was large and awkwardly designed. It wasn't long before her pain returned. "I developed shooting pains in my left hand," Shelly recalled. "Just touching the computer keyboard was painful." The new diagnosis: carpal tunnel syndrome.

Debbie worked as a cashier in a supermarket. Every day, for hours on end, she would pass items over a computer scanner for a readout of the price. Sometimes the price wouldn't appear immediately—she'd twist the item this way and that, trying to get the computer to "see" it. She did this with everything, from jars of baby food to half-gallon bottles of juice. If two or three attempts were unsuccessful, she'd give up entirely and punch in the price in the old-fashioned way.

Debbie's pain started at night, shooting through her left hand and wrist. Often the pain would wake her up, and her hands would be swollen in the morning. Her doctor gave her hand braces to wear to bed. Her only comfortable sleeping position was on her back, with her hands crossed over her chest—"just as if I was in a coffin," she said. She began losing strength in her left hand. The doctor's diagnosis: carpal tunnel syndrome.

There's nothing mysterious about carpal tunnel syndrome (CTS). As you'll learn in the chapters to come, it happens when you twist or bend your wrist repeatedly. Done often enough, this movement causes the coverings of the tendons in the fingers and hand to swell and press on a nerve called the median nerve, which passes through a portion of the wrist known as the carpal tunnel. CTS may also arise when you hold your wrist in an awkward position for hours on end, which you may do if you work at a computer keyboard.

Carpal tunnel syndrome doesn't happen after one awkward movement, the way a sprain or a ligament tear does. It results from doing the same wrist movements hour after hour, day after day. For example Debbie the cashier lifted heavy objects over her computer scanner continually during every eight-hour shift. Often she'd have to pass the same item over the scanner several times to get a readout. People who hold wrenches or drills all the time also develop CTS; in fact anyone whose job requires her to flex or extend her wrist constantly is vulnerable to carpal tunnel syndrome. Along with pain in one or both hands and arms, the symptoms may include loss of feeling in portions of the hand and tingling or a "pins and needles" sensation in the thumb, index and middle fingers, and part of the ring finger.

As you'll learn in subsequent chapters, the diagnosis and treatment of CTS are straightforward. Milder cases readily respond to therapy, but more severe cases may leave patients unable to write a note, drive a car, clean their homes, shop, or even comb their hair. That's why it's important to learn about the syndrome's early symptoms and seek treatment promptly.

Doctors have known about carpal tunnel syndrome for over a hundred years. It was first formally noted in 1865, when the British physician Sir James Paget described a wrist fracture that resulted in compression of the median nerve. But carpal tunnel syndrome was thought to be relatively rare until the last few decades. Since then it has become one of the most common conditions treated by hand surgeons. According to one national survey, in one year four hundred hand surgeons performed 26,000 operations to correct carpal tunnel syndrome. Some experts estimate that the actual figure may be closer to 100,000 operations annually.

Why the recent explosion of carpal tunnel syndrome? Most likely because of the revolution in the modern workplace. There were 675,000 video display terminals (commonly referred to as VDTs) in the American workplace in 1976; by the mid-1990s, there will be about 80 million. As the use of VDTs has grown, so has the incidence of carpal tunnel syndrome. There are many reasons why this has occurred, but one of the most important is that VDTs have cut down on the diversity of office work. Typing, filing, and interoffice communication were once separate tasks involving very different activities, but today many office workers type documents, keep files, and communicate with other employees all through their computer terminals. The result: hour upon hour at the VDT, doing the same limited repertoire of motions all the time. Add to this the often awkward design of keyboards and workstations, and you have a situation ripe for the development of carpal tunnel syndrome.

Nor does CTS result only from using video display terminals. Meat packers, fish filleters, automobile assemblers, and even sign-language interpreters are among the long list of workers who risk developing CTS. Greater automation of the workplace has, in many instances, led to greater specialization of duties, so that one employee may perform only a few tasks thousands of times a day, using the same wrist motion each time. In fact CTS is but one of a group of conditions that arise from repeating the same awkward movement over and over again. Known by several names—repetitive motion disorders, cumulative trauma disorders, and repetitive strain injuries, to name a few—these syndromes are proliferating as the demands of the workplace are given precedence over the needs of the human body. In this book we'll call these conditions repetitive motion disorders, or RMDs.

Whatever you call them, these diseases are among the leading causes of occupational illness. According to the Bureau of Labor Statistics, repeated traumas constituted 48 percent of the 240,900 occupational illnesses reported in 1988—that's 115,400 cases, up 10 percent from the year before. Others have estimated that some

20 million people have jobs with a significant risk of developing an RMD. In one study conducted at an athletic products plant, 35.8 percent of the workers tested had an RMD reimbursable by workers' compensation. And in a nationwide survey conducted by the Communications Workers of America, the union that represents telephone operators, 30 to 60 percent of the 12,000 respondents reported suffering from RMDs. The American Academy of Orthopedic Surgeons estimates that RMDs cost industry more than $27 billion each year in lost earnings and medical expenses. As recently as June 16, 1990, eight journalists filed a $270 million suit in federal court against a manufacturer of word processing equipment for newspapers. According to the suit, these workers have developed several RMDs from using that particular system.

Troubled by the growing incidence of RMDs, the House of Representatives conducted hearings on the problem in 1989, through the Employment and Housing Subcommittee of the Committee on Government Operations. According to the subcommittee's chairman, Tom Lantos (D-California), carpal tunnel syndrome and the other RMDs may be the occupational hazard of the nineties. "Unfortunately I anticipate an increase of these disorders in at least the early years of the 1990s with increased use of video display terminals, computerized checkout scanners, and other equipment which is responsible for the problem," he says. He adds, however, that greater awareness of these conditions, coupled with stricter enforcement of workplace regulations by the Occupational Safety and Health Administration (OSHA) and the National Institute of Occupational Safety and Health

(NIOSH), should elicit improvements as the decade wears on.

According to a report from NIOSH, carpal tunnel syndrome is currently three to ten times more common in women than men—probably due, at least in part, to the activity of female hormones, as you'll learn in the first chapter. It's rarely seen before the age of sixteen and is most common between the ages of thirty and seventy, prompting some experts to describe carpal tunnel syndrome as a disease of middle age. But this profile is changing as more and more work-related cases occur. The number of men under thirty with carpal tunnel syndrome is rising. According to NIOSH estimates, 15 to 20 percent of all workers in construction, mining, clerical, and food preparation jobs are at risk of developing RMDs such as carpal tunnel syndrome.

Many industries now list CTS among their most costly and disabling medical problems. A single case of CTS may cost a company as much as $25,000 in lost work time, medical costs, and permanent partial disability awards. In one meat-packing plant alone, days lost from work and workers' compensation claims due to CTS totaled more than $1 million between 1981 and 1986. For each hand affected, an average of fifty-four days were lost from work, and the average compensation settlement was over $8,000, not including hospital costs and doctors' fees. At one point the workers' compensation claims due to CTS were so costly and numerous that the plant's managers considered shutting down.

So carpal tunnel syndrome is very much a disorder of the late-twentieth-century workplace. But it does not result only from work. Anything that compresses the median nerve during its journey through the wrist may lead to carpal tunnel syndrome. Thus certain kinds of trauma, such as a wrist fracture, or conditions that affect nerve function, such as diabetes, may place you at risk of developing carpal tunnel syndrome, as might a sport or hobby that requires repeated motion of the wrist. What's more, people often have more than one RMD at a time, making correct diagnosis and treatment especially crucial.

Nevertheless the recent increase in carpal tunnel syndrome and similar disorders is due almost entirely to the changing nature of the workplace. To understand fully the development, treatment, and prevention of carpal tunnel syndrome, you must also know something about modern-day work and the options available to employees. In this book you'll learn about the medical aspects of carpal tunnel syndrome and other RMDs—what they are, how they develop, how doctors diagnose and treat them. You'll find that carpal tunnel syndrome has certain classic signs and symptoms that make it relatively easy for an experienced doctor to recognize. Some of the related RMDs also have distinctive symptoms, but others may appear simply as pain in the hand or wrist, with no signs that can be objectively measured. In these cases doctor and patient must work together to relate the symptoms to a particular activity.

But you'll also learn that sometimes the only way of treating these disorders or of preventing their recurrence is to change the way you work. In this case one way you can protect your health is to learn about your rights as an employee.

In chapter 1 you'll learn how your hands work and

what makes them vulnerable to conditions such as carpal tunnel syndrome. Chapter 2 explains how doctors diagnose carpal tunnel syndrome and other RMDs, chiefly through studying your symptoms and employing special tests. Chapter 3 covers the treatment of these conditions.

Chapter 4 introduces you to the best hope of eliminating RMDs: the science of ergonomics. Experts in this discipline are studying ways of providing you with a safer, more comfortable workplace. You'll also discover which jobs may be hazardous to your health and what you can do to improve your working conditions. If your employer resists your efforts to make workplace changes, chapter 5 shows you how you can enlist the aid of government agencies—and why it's in your company's financial interest to respond before you take that step. In chapter 6 you'll find out where to get more information about CTS and related disorders in general, about your rights in the workplace, and about how to proceed with legal or government action.

Carpal tunnel syndrome is simple to diagnose and treat. But while few cases are severe enough to cause permanent disability, patients may pay dearly in terms of pain, inconvenience, emotional distress, and time lost from work. The more you know about CTS, the better you can protect yourself.

WHAT IS CARPAL TUNNEL SYNDROME?

What would you do without your hands?

You wouldn't be able to turn the pages of this book. You wouldn't be able to cook a meal, drive to work, diaper a baby, pet a dog, comb your hair, apply makeup, tie a tie, make your bed, fix a flat tire, write a letter, or tie your shoes. You wouldn't be able to scratch an itch, blow your nose, or even feed yourself. In fact you can probably think of dozens, possibly hundreds, of other tasks you perform with your hands, day in and day out, that you've never considered before. Try to imagine what life would be like if you couldn't use your hands and you'll have some idea of what it's like for those with the pain and disability of carpal tunnel syndrome (CTS). If you've ever had CTS or some other affliction of the hands, you know this already—firsthand.

A HAND FOR YOUR HANDS

Your hands are composed of muscles, nerves, tendons, ligaments, and twenty-seven delicate bones that all work together with the precision of a fine watch.

The human hand contains two kinds of muscles: flexors and extensors. Running from the hands down the front of the forearms, flexor muscles are responsible for flexing the fingers and the wrist, for closing a fist, and for bending the hand down. Extensor muscles travel down the back of the forearm and allow you to extend your wrist and fingers, open your fist, and bend your hand backward. Want to move your hand from side to side? The flexors and extensors work together to bend your hand toward your pinky or your thumb. Tendons connect these muscles to the finger bones and help transmit the strength of muscular force when a strong grip is required.

Also crucial to hand function are the nerves. Three major nerves feed the hand and ultimately connect with cells in the spinal cord and brain, allowing you to pull your hand away from a painful stimulus or perform a fine movement, such as playing the harp. Of these three, one figures prominently in the development of CTS: the median nerve.

Originating in the spinal cord, the median nerve courses down the arm and through the wrist. It branches out in the hand to supply the thumb, forefinger, middle finger, and half of the ring finger. In fact it's this unique distribution of the median nerve that gives CTS its distinctive symptoms. Doctors sometimes call the median nerve the eye of the hand because it's so important to

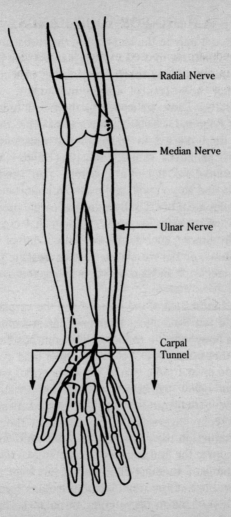

Radial Nerve

Median Nerve

Ulnar Nerve

Carpal Tunnel

Figure 1. The median nerve runs through the arm and hand.

hand function: It helps maintain the flexors and other muscles, not only in the hand but in the forearm as well.

If you could see into your wrist, just where it joins the palm, you would see the median nerve, plus nine tendons that help control finger movement, traveling through a bony passage known as the carpal tunnel. The tunnel's floor and walls are composed of bone (the carpal bones); its roof is a rigid ligament—the transverse carpal ligament, or flexor retinaculum—that binds the wrist joint, helps the tendons generate the hand's grip strength, and as you will see, plays an important role in the development of CTS. Because the carpal tunnel is so narrow and its walls so rigid, anything that crowds the space even more, such as the swelling of one or more of the tendons, or the membrane that covers the tendons, may squeeze the median nerve, creating the symptoms of CTS.

For a better idea of the structure of the carpal tunnel, hold your left hand about twelve inches in front of you. Feel the bony junction of the back of your hand and your wrist—these are the carpal bones. Now hold your hand palm side up and place two or three fingers of your right hand just below the crease of your left wrist. Slowly open and close your left fist. The movement you feel beneath your fingers is the movement of the tendons that run through the carpal tunnel. And when you move your fingers, the tendons rub against the walls of the carpal tunnel, something like a belt sliding over a pulley. Together the median nerve and the tendons form a bundle, with the median nerve going through the middle of the bundle and the transverse carpal ligament binding it together. Figure 1 shows the median nerve and its relationship to other structures in the arm and wrist; figure 2 presents a cross-sectional, right-handed view of the carpal tunnel and the structures it contains. In figure 3 you see the carpal tunnel as you would if you were looking into the palm of the right hand.

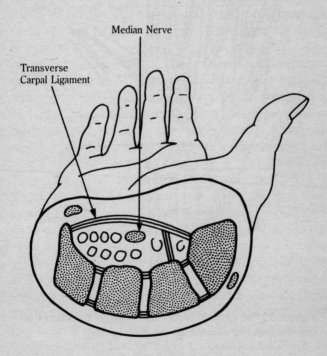

Figure 2. A cross-sectional view of the carpal tunnel and some of its structures in the right wrist.

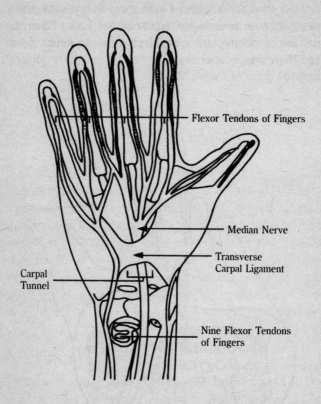

Flexor Tendons of Fingers

Median Nerve

Transverse
Carpal Ligament

Carpal
Tunnel

Nine Flexor Tendons
of Fingers

Figure 3. The carpal tunnel and related structures as viewed looking down into the right palm.

The wrist is the hand's key joint. It governs finger movement as well as movement of the entire hand. So it's not surprising that a problem with the wrist affects hand function as a whole.

HOW CARPAL TUNNEL SYNDROME DEVELOPS

As mentioned in the introduction, most cases of CTS seen today occur when the same motion is performed again and again, day in and day out, over the course of several months or years. That's why CTS is so frequently related to work. The essential factor here is repetition. Doing something once or twice, or even one hundred times, won't lead to CTS. The problem occurs when you perform the same limited assortment of tasks repeatedly—on the job or as part of certain hobbies or sports.

As you've seen, movement of the hand or fingers causes the associated tendons to slide against the walls of the carpal tunnel. Done often enough, this movement will irritate the tendons, or their coverings, making them swollen and inflamed. There's nowhere for these swollen tendons to go in the already crowded carpal tunnel, so they press against other tunnel structures—most notably the median nerve. What is worse is that, along with repetition, so many jobs require hand positions that are awkward or uncomfortable. There is some evidence that extreme flexion or extension of the fingers or wrist raises pressure within the carpal tunnel, possibly hastening the irritation of the tendons.

The position of greatest hand comfort and efficiency is sometimes called the position of function: with the elbow bent as if for working at a table or desk, the wrist is extended slightly upward, about 30 degrees, and the fingers are loosely curled. This position favors the strongest grip or pinch with the least likelihood of fatigue.

Probably the most awkward position is the position of rest: Again the elbow is bent, but this time the wrist is flexed so that the hands hang down and the fingers are extended. Try doing something with your hands in this position—you'll probably find that you can't generate your usual grip or pinch strength, and your hands or arms may tire more quickly than normal. People who work with their hands in this position, or a less extreme variation of it, all the time run the greatest risk of developing CTS.

SYMPTOMS OF CARPAL TUNNEL SYNDROME

It takes time for CTS to develop. And once CTS sets in, it often has time to worsen because few people recognize their initial symptoms as early CTS. Instead they may chalk them up to a sprain or strain, poor circulation, or the arm or hand having "fallen asleep."

The most common symptoms of CTS reflect the median nerve's distribution in the hand. They include:

- **Pain.** The wrist, palm, thumb, and index, middle, and part of the ring finger are all served by the median nerve. Pain may occur in any or all of these areas and extend up the forearm, sometimes all the way up to the shoulder. In the condition's early stages patients experience these symptoms at night, often after they've gone to bed. Frequently the pain wakes them.

- **Tingling or numbness in the fingers or palm.** Many patients describe the sensation as burning, aching, or pricking. Some people say their fingers feel useless and swollen, even if the fingers don't look swollen to an impartial observer. Along with the pain these symptoms are often worst in the fingertips.

- **Clumsiness of the hand.** Once again, median-nerve impairment is the culprit behind this symptom.

- **Wasting of the muscle at the base of the thumb.** This muscle, called the thenar muscle, may deteriorate if the CTS has gone untreated for several years. Here again, dysfunction of the median nerve is the true culprit and contributes to the clumsiness.

The Progression of CTS

As mentioned above, the earliest symptoms of CTS typically begin slowly and are mistaken for something else. A person's hands may feel tired, or her wrists may feel sore. The first indications may also be a feeling of numbness, tingling, or "pins and needles." These symptoms start after work or later at night, after the patient has gone to bed, because it's during sleep that blood may collect in the small blood vessels feeding the damaged tissue in the hand, leading to swelling of those vessels and pressure on the median nerve. Also, people tend to sleep with their wrists flexed. Many people find relief through shaking or rubbing their hands, which gets the blood flowing again and restores the wrist to a neutral position. Pain may or may not be present in the disease's beginning stages.

As CTS progresses, these symptoms slowly become stronger and more persistent, until you feel them all the time. Sometimes other signs of nerve damage appear, most likely a loss of hand strength or sensation, but these don't occur in all patients and even when they do, it's usually after the other symptoms have been present for years. People may tolerate the discomfort of CTS for months or even years before seeking help because it takes that long for them to realize that their condition is really abnormal. If CTS is allowed to exist long enough without treatment, the median nerve and thenar muscle may atrophy, leading to permanent loss of hand sensation or strength. Some people also lose the ability to distinguish between hot and cold in the affected hand.

In short, median-nerve damage diminishes the hand's ability to detect an object's sensory qualities—its weight, for example, or shape, as well as its temperature. This loss of sensory feedback affects your ability to grasp, hold, or manipulate objects because the hand lacks the appropriate information and cannot assume the proper position or generate the right amount of strength, all of which it normally does with little if any consciousness on your part. Thus the clumsiness that comes with

CTS develops for two reasons: first, a genuine loss of strength due to muscular atrophy; and second, the inability to obtain the right sensory information about the object in question.

Atypical Symptoms of CTS

Occasionally people with CTS develop some unexpected symptoms: swelling of the underside of the wrist due to inflammation of the flexor tendon (one of the tendons occupying the carpal tunnel); pain in the elbow or shoulder; and excessive sweating, dryness, or shininess of the palm due to impairment of the sweat glands, also a result of nerve damage. This last symptom may also contribute to the clumsiness associated with CTS, because the palm's moisture plays an important role in generating the friction necessary to grasp and manipulate things. Other symptoms sometimes associated with CTS include color changes in the fingers, as well as mild water retention, known as edema, in the fingers or hand.

Other Causes of CTS

While most of the cases of CTS doctors see today are related to awkward, repetitive movements on the job, it has other causes as well. Essentially any condition that affects nerve conduction may lead to CTS. The syndrome has been associated with several medical conditions, including:

- Diabetes

- Rheumatoid arthritis

- An underactive thyroid, a condition known as myxedema

- Kidney failure

- Prolonged alcoholism

- Certain forms of cancer that might lead to tumors in the wrist

- Rare congenital disorders, such as protrusions of muscle or bone into the wrist, or defects of the median nerve

Pregnancy also seems to increase the risk of CTS in some women. Some doctors think this may be due to changes in hormonal activity, which may lead to water retention and swelling of the tissues in the carpal tunnel. CTS has been related to some sports as well, such as:

- **Weight lifting.** For weight lifters the source of the problem seems to be the bands they wrap around their wrists for support. When wrapped too tightly, the bands place pressure on the wrist and the carpal tunnel. Weight lifters and body builders who use wrist bands should make sure they fit comfortably and use them more as a reminder to keep the wrist straight, as should anyone who engages in the other activities listed.

- **Racquet sports.** People who engage in sports such as racquetball, which is played in an enclosed court, use their flexed wrists to wield the racquet and to help them bounce back when they hit the walls during play. For frequent players this may place intolerable stress on the wrist.

- **Swimming.** When lap swimmers reach the end of the pool, they often hit the pool's wall or grab it briefly and push off from it as they start the next lap. Done often enough, this may irritate wrist tendons and lead to the development of CTS.

- **Running.** It may seem surprising that running could affect one's wrists, but many runners make tight fists or open and close their hands while exercising. Hand weights exacerbate the problem.

- **Aerobics.** Here again hand weights are the source of injury. When too heavy they cause the hand to flex forward to accommodate the weight, placing strain on the wrists. If you must use hand weights during aerobics, make sure they're light enough for you to use comfortably.

- **Exercise machines.** Exercise bikes, rowing machines, or stair-climbers may all figure in the development of CTS. The wrist contributes to the action in rowing and bike machines, and the continual flexion and extension may irritate tendons in the carpal tunnel. On the stair-climbing machine, many people compensate for increasing speed by leaning on the hand rails, forcing the wrist into an unnatural position that may lead to irritation of the tendons in the wrist.

Role of Wrist Size

In an effort to identify those who might run a higher-than-average risk of developing CTS, some researchers have suggested that people with unusually small wrists might be especially vulnerable. But so far no one has found any conclusive evidence that wrist size influences your risk of CTS. Most experts believe there is no relationship.

CONCLUSION

The symptoms of CTS are usually pretty consistent from one patient to the next, so the right doctor can diagnose it fairly quickly. Nevertheless some challenges do exist. As mentioned earlier, many people live with this condition for months or years before seeking help. By the time they consult a doctor, the CTS may be in an advanced stage, sometimes with permanent damage to the median nerve or thenar muscle. And CTS often occurs with other repetitive motion disorders of the hand, elbow, or shoulder, all of which may have similar symptoms. Thus the doctor may treat one of the other problems, only to realize later that the patient has CTS as well.

The good news is that carpal tunnel syndrome readily responds to therapy when it's caught and treated promptly. Chapter 2 tells you what's involved in diagnosing carpal tunnel syndrome and other RMDs and how to find a doctor who can do that for you. In chapter 3 you'll learn how these conditions are treated.

HELPING HANDS: DIAGNOSING REPETITIVE MOTION DISORDERS

Okay, your hand hurts. Maybe your fingers ache; maybe it's your palm. Or maybe the pain is more in your elbow or forearm, instead of your hands. Perhaps what you're feeling isn't really pain; it's more like a tingling, or numbness, or the "pins and needles" feeling you get when a limb "goes to sleep."

As explained in chapter 1, any or all of these may be symptoms of carpal tunnel syndrome. But they may signal other disorders as well. In fact it's not uncommon for people to develop several RMDs together, for the circumstances that promote one promote several. Therefore it's worthwhile taking a closer look at RMDs in general.

Repetitive motion disorders are disorders of the muscle and skeletal system related to damage to tendons and/or the sheaths that cover them and to related bones, muscles, and nerves. In this book we concentrate on

RMDs of the hand and wrist, but these disorders may also appear in the feet, knees, or back. As mentioned in the introduction, RMDs may have other names. Many people refer to them simply as overuse injuries because they result when the body's healing or adaptive powers cannot keep up with the demands of the situation, as, for example, when you perform the same set of motions day after day on a job. RMDs develop slowly and result from repeated actions, unlike an injury that comes from an accident or some other brief event.

Two or more RMDs may occur simultaneously due to the number of muscles and nerves in the hand and the precision with which they interact. For example many vibrating tools, such as power drills, must be held at an awkward angle with bent wrists and require a significant amount of force to hold them upright and work them properly. All of these conditions—strong vibration, wrist bent in an awkward position, and the exertion of force—are associated with the development of RMDs.

Perhaps one reason why so many people hesitate to link RMDs with work is that it's hard to understand how an activity that's harmless for a few minutes can cause so much damage when it's done over and over again. For a bit of insight as to how this might occur, go find the least comfortable chair in your office or home and sit there, in the same position, for fifteen minutes. Go on, try it.

How did it feel? Chances are it was all right for the first five minutes or so, but after that you probably started to feel uncomfortable. Maybe your back or your rear end started to hurt, or perhaps you got a restless feeling in your legs. No doubt you soon wanted to shift your position; perhaps you did so without even realizing it.

You felt these sensations because, by sitting in one position for more than a few minutes, you restricted the flow of blood through the muscles in that part of your body. Normally muscle cells manufacture metabolic waste products that can be carried away in the blood when it flows freely, but when circulation is limited, the waste products accumulate in the muscle tissue, leading to the aches and discomfort associated with fatigue and immobility.

How is this related to repetitive motion? Suppose your job requires you to sit in essentially the same position, hour after hour, performing the same group of tasks over and over again. Over the short term, as your discomfort mounts, you may be more and more easily distracted from your work. Perhaps you make more mistakes, or your productivity declines, or you have a few accidents. Nevertheless you may still find relief through rest or a change in activity. But ultimately there comes a point when long-term damage sets in, through the buildup of metabolic wastes in the muscles and tendons and through the inflammation resulting from the strain of repetitive motion and an awkward position. At this point you may feel pain after only brief periods of work— indeed for some people the pain is constant—and rest is less likely to bring relief. You've crossed that elusive line from discomfort to disease.

SYMPTOMS OF REPETITIVE MOTION DISORDERS

Repetitive motion disorders share certain symptoms: pain, aching, and/or burning sensations that radiate from the affected area to nearby parts of the body. For example pain from an RMD in the hand may radiate up the forearm to the elbow and perhaps even the shoulder. Other symptoms include:

- Swelling of the affected area

- Jerky movements of the joint, or a snapping sound—known as crepitus—when you move the affected joint

- Nodules that form on tendons

- A positive response to Finkelstein's test, described in the section on diagnostic tests

Repetitive motion disorders also have certain characteristics in common. They

- Correspond to the intensity of the work

- Involve biomechanical and physiological mechanisms

- May occur after weeks, months, or years on the job, and they may require weeks, months, or even years to subside completely

- Have both occupational and nonoccupational causes

- May have poorly localized, nonspecific symptoms

It's this last quality that has made RMDs so difficult to diagnose, and employers so reluctant to admit that they might be work related. As stated in the introduction, an RMD may appear as nothing more than aching or tingling in the hand, wrist, or arm. It may appear at night or while the person is resting, making it difficult to relate to one's job. What's more, few if any studies exist that have investigated the effects of making changes in the workplaces of people who already have RMDs, or how these changes affect the incidence of new cases. Do changes in the workplace give relief to those already suffering? Do they protect others from developing RMDs? The actual statistics have yet to be compiled, even though common sense might say yes to both questions. In fact people have instinctively associated certain problems with work for centuries. Old medical texts contain references to disorders such as "washerwoman's hands" or "gamekeeper's thumb"; today these are known as de-Quervain's syndrome or tenosynovitis.

Fortunately the risk of permanent damage from an RMD is slight—*if* you detect it and treat it in time. For many reasons people often ignore their symptoms and continue the activity responsible for their woes until it's too late. A prompt, accurate diagnosis is essential to effective treatment, and for that you need a doctor experienced in treating disorders of the hand.

FINDING THE RIGHT DOCTOR

Many doctors take a special interest in diseases of the hand: orthopedists, plastic surgeons, general surgeons, neurologists, sports-medicine specialists, and rheumatologists all treat hand disorders. Many do so on a regular basis, and some even specialize exclusively in hand problems.

Whomever you choose, the qualities you investigate should include his or her experience in treating hand conditions, as well as the personal "chemistry" that exists between you. Even with many years' experience and a wallful of degrees, a doctor with whom you don't feel comfortable is probably not the doctor for you.

Your general or family practitioner may be able to refer you to a good hand specialist. If that isn't possible, call a local hospital and ask if they can refer you, or, if your community has a medical school, contact the surgery or orthopedics department for a list of faculty members who see private patients. Local television stations in some cities advertise doctor referral services. You may indeed be able to find a good physician through one of these organizations, but keep in mind that the doctors pay to be listed with them; there's usually little if any screening involved. Finally chapter 6 contains a list of organizations of medical specialists; you might contact them and ask for the names of physicians in your area.

Here's a list of questions you may want to keep in mind as you look for a doctor:

- Is he board-qualified and certified in his particular specialty? If so, he has had to meet certain standards of training and practice and has passed an exam to receive certification.

- Has he completed an intensive fellowship in hand disorders? You would want to know this particularly about a young doctor.

• What percentage of his practice is currently composed of hand cases? Experience is important to a good outcome. If a doctor says he specializes in hand problems, such cases should comprise at least 15 percent of his practice.

DIAGNOSING CARPAL TUNNEL SYNDROME AND OTHER RMDS

In diagnosing your problem, your doctor will most likely rely on the medical history and the physical examination, which together form the foundation of good medical practice. The descriptions that follow emphasize the diagnosis of carpal tunnel syndrome, but as you'll see, many of the tests can be used to detect other RMDs as well.

Medical History

Many doctors believe that an accurate medical history is the best indicator of an RMD. During your examination the doctor will ask about your age, your dominant hand, your occupation, and any previous history of hand problems. In the occupational history he'll probably want to know more about the tasks you perform with your hands, how often you perform them each day, and how long you've had your job. He may also ask you about hobbies, sports, and other activities that involve the use of your hands, and about other medical conditions such as thyroid problems or diabetes.

Physical Examination

Next the doctor will examine your hands themselves. He'll check for pain and nerve sensitivity; most likely he'll also test your reflexes and may check for evidence of muscle wasting. In addition he'll observe the function of your neck, shoulders, and upper arms, watching for any signs of pain or limitation on their normal range of motion.

During the examination the doctor will probably evaluate your hand function by having you reach for the ceiling, open and close your fists, and touch your thumb to each fingertip in sequence. If you have carpal tunnel syndrome, the physical exam will probably reveal pain or sensory disturbances (for example numbness or tingling) restricted to that portion of the hand served by the median nerve—thumb, index, and middle fingers on the palm side; the first half of the ring finger on the palm side; and the back (dorsal) side of all of those fingers down to the middle joint; also the first half of the palm. To confirm the diagnosis of carpal tunnel syndrome or some other RMD, he may conduct one or more of the following tests:

Phalen's test (also known as Phalen's sign).   For this test, considered one of the most valuable clinical signs of CTS, the doctor will have you flex your wrist tightly for thirty to sixty seconds, compressing the median nerve. This is usually done by putting the backs of your hands together, causing a sharp flexion in each wrist. People with CTS will experience the pain and other symptoms associated with the syndrome in the affected hand. However while Phalen's test is considered an important test for the presence of CTS, it does not detect all cases. In some studies it has been positive in as few as 40 percent of the people who had CTS.

Tinel's sign. To elicit Tinel's sign, the doctor will gently tap your wrist. The sign is present if you feel tingling or pain in one or more fingers in response. Some experts claim that Tinel's sign may be less common in CTS patients than previously thought; it may occur in only 60 percent of people with the condition. In one experiment on people known to have CTS, investigators found Tinel's sign in only 28 percent of the subjects.

Weakness or atrophy of hand muscles. Muscles contract in response to signals from nerves, so when a nerve is damaged, the muscles served by that nerve may deteriorate. This is what happens in some instances of CTS, especially those that have gone untreated for a long time. Wasting of a hand muscle known as the abductor pollicis brevis, which bends the thumb and pulls it away from the other fingers, often indicates the presence of CTS.

Improvement following injection of steroids and lidocaine into the carpal tunnel. As you'll see in the chapter on treatment, steroid injections are a standard therapy for mild-to-moderate cases of carpal tunnel syndrome and other RMDs. They relieve the tendon inflammation associated with the condition and thus much of the pain and other symptoms. Lidocaine is a mild anesthetic, so it, too, helps relieve pain.

OTHER METHODS OF DIAGNOSIS

An experienced physician can diagnose most cases of CTS using the methods just described. However there are always those cases in which several conditions may be present simultaneously, or the results of the usual tests are inconclusive, or the symptoms just aren't clear. And even among patients whose CTS is easily diagnosed, there are those who require documentation for insurance claims or workers' compensation. All of these people need tests that doctors normally hesitate to perform because they're elaborate or expensive and don't necessarily yield more information than the simpler tests. But sometimes they're useful, and a physician may use them when he has questions about a case.

Electrodiagnostic Techniques

More commonly known as electromyography nerve conduction velocity (EMG/NCV), electrodiagnostic techniques measure the electrical activity of the muscles and nerves in question. An oscilloscope displays the results, which may be photographed or recorded on special tape for a permanent record. In testing for CTS, the investigator places surface electrodes over the median nerve in the wrist. In the index finger he inserts needle electrodes, which may be painful. He'll then stimulate nerve activity in the finger and record the response in the median nerve. Surface electrodes over the base of the thumb detect electrical activity in the abductor pollicis brevis muscle following stimulation of the median nerve with the electrodes attached to the wrist. Electrodes may also be applied to the forearm and the speed of nerve impulses measured from there to the wrist or thumb.

The idea behind these tests is to measure the time it takes for impulses to travel from one part of the median nerve to another, or from the nerve to one of its muscles. These impulses usually move more slowly with CTS, but a small but significant number of patients with CTS exhibit a normal response to EMG/NCV. NCV is probably best used to help distinguish between CTS and other nerve problems, or, since it may provide a permanent, objective record, for those people who require proof of their condition (providing, of course, the test detects their CTS). Because it also measures muscle tension under various circumstances, EMG may also play a role in the creation of better-designed tools that decrease the worker's risk of developing CTS.

Vibration Sensation

People with CTS often lose some of their ability to detect vibration with the affected hand, because some of the nerve fibers that respond to this sensation may deteriorate. Thus measurement of vibration perception, using an instrument called a vibrometer, is another possible test for CTS. The vibrometer assesses vibration perception in the index finger, which is fed by the median nerve, and compares it to vibration perception in the little finger in the same hand, which is fed by a different nerve (the ulnar nerve). Loss of vibration perception in the index finger is a good signal of early CTS.

Like EMG, the vibrometer may provide documentation of the condition for those who need it, only without the pain and at less expense.

Arthroscopy

An arthroscope is a specially designed tube with a light at one end that may be inserted into a joint through a small incision. The doctor then peers into the arthroscope for a firsthand view of the joint's condition. The knees are the most common targets of arthroscopy, but some doctors use it occasionally for an inside view of the wrist in cases of CTS.

Arthrogram

For a picture of what's going on in the wrist, a doctor may take a special X ray known as an arthrogram by injecting a contrast medium into the wrist and photographing it.

Computerized (Computed) Tomography

Usually referred to as CT, this technique employs a computer to scan the body, or parts of it, in sections, permitting a three-dimensional view of structures that may previously have been hidden or only partially visible. When diagnosing carpal tunnel syndrome, some doctors have used CT to see if there is anything in the carpal tunnel that might be pressing on the median nerve, such as:

• A fat deposit in the wrist (this is an abnormal condition, unrelated to body weight)

• A protrusion of muscle or bone into the tunnel

• A previously undetected wrist fracture

• Thickening of the transverse carpal ligament, which runs through the carpal tunnel

Tourniquet Test

The "tourniquet" used in this test is a common blood pressure cuff, which is placed on your arm and inflated, putting pressure on the median nerve. If you have CTS, you'll start to feel pain and tingling as the cuff is tightened. The tourniquet test is considered even less accurate than the wrist flexion (Phalen's) test, so it is used less frequently.

X rays

X rays are a standard part of the examination.

Finger Symptoms

One very simple way to discover if your symptoms are the result of CTS or of something else is to concentrate on your pinky. Does it, too, feel painful or numb? If so, you don't have CTS (or you have something else along with CTS), because median-nerve compression never causes symptoms in the little finger. Similarly, you don't have CTS if your symptoms don't occur in at least one of the first three fingers (thumb, index, or middle finger); these are the fingers innervated most extensively by the median nerve.

The Do-It-Yourself Test

Most doctors cringe at the thought of patients diagnosing themselves, but in fact there is a crude do-it-yourself test for those who suspect they may have CTS. Make a fist and hold it, without exerting undue pressure, for thirty to sixty seconds. If you start feeling pain or tingling in that hand, it is possible that you have CTS. Seek medical help immediately, but don't panic—just remember that the test *is* crude, and far from foolproof.

DIAGNOSING THE OTHER RMDS

As noted above, some RMDs have vague, nonspecific symptoms, such as pain, tingling, or numbness in the fingers, hand, or wrist. There are, however, some easily identified RMDs that may be diagnosed from their characteristic symptoms. Among these disorders are:

Tenosynovitis (or Synovitis)

This is the name for inflammation of a tendon, along with its covering membrane, known as the synovium or synovial sheath. Extreme flexion or side-to-side movement of the joint is especially liable to cause tenosynovitis, but this condition may have other causes, unrelated to work or repetitive motion, as well: gout, gonorrhea, calcium deposits in the wrist, or rheumatoid arthritis. It's also been associated with sports such as crew (rowing) or basketball, which require a lot of wrist action.

Theoretically tenosynovitis is not limited to tendons of the hand or wrist. However tenosynovitis in this part of the body is one of the most common of the RMDs. What's more, the word *tenosynovitis* may refer to the inflammation of a specific tendon, or it may be used to describe a whole group of disorders. For example carpal tunnel syndrome is considered a form of tenosynovitis, as is that disorder known as trigger finger, which is discussed in more detail below.

Symptoms of tenosynovitis include pain during any motion in the afflicted finger or wrist, which may ultimately become serious enough to prevent the patient from working. People with tenosynovitis may also experience swelling or crepitus along the wrist tendons and up the arm, as well as tenderness in the tendon area. A thorough medical history and physical examination are usually sufficient for a doctor to diagnose tenosynovitis.

Trigger Finger

This form of tenosynovitis occurs when the finger is flexed frequently against resistance, as it might be if you were pulling a trigger repeatedly. Eventually the tendon and synovial sheath in that finger may swell, and a nodule may form on the tendon, interfering with finger movement.

The symptoms of trigger finger are often most noticeable in the morning. Your movements during the day help prevent blood from accumulating in any one place for too long, but when you're asleep, blood may collect in certain tissues, including those of the hand. Add to this the flexed position normally assumed by the hands during sleep, and an inflamed tendon, or the tissues around it, may swell so much that someone with this condition may wake up to find her finger caught in the flexed position. At first extension of the finger may be too painful, but then the finger may suddenly "snap" into the extended position and be locked there. Similarly the patient may be unable to flex her finger, until it snaps into a flexed position and remains locked. Often finger movement becomes easier as the day wears on and the pooled fluid has a chance to move out of the tissues.

This "snapping" and "locking" phenomenon is characteristic of trigger finger and may be diagnostic for the condition in its earlier stages. In more advanced cases weakening of the extensor muscles may make it harder to extend than to flex the finger, and some patients find that they can extend the finger only by pulling it with the other hand. In the most extreme cases the finger becomes locked in the flexed or extended position and cannot be moved at all.

DeQuervain's Syndrome

Named for the Swiss doctor who first described it in 1895, this form of tenosynovitis (sometimes called De-Quervaine's or deQuervain's disease) consists of inflammation and swelling of the tendons running down the base and the back of the thumb, into the wrist. De-Quervain's syndrome results from the friction between the tendon, its sheath, and the bone generated by pinching the thumb and simultaneously moving the wrist, especially flexing it. The condition is especially common among women who perform repetitive, manual tasks that involve inward hand motion and a strong grip.

Symptoms of deQuervain's syndrome include aching at the outside base of the thumb, where it joins the wrist, into the small compartment you can feel just above your wrist joint and just below the base of the thumb. The pain may radiate into the hand or even the forearm. One of the diagnostic tests a doctor may use is to have you flex your thumb so that it sits in your palm just under your fingers. With the thumb in this position, he'll ask you to bend your hand toward your pinky. This motion stretches the thumb tendons and may reproduce your symptoms if you have deQuervain's syndrome. Alternatively he may ask you to flex your thumb outward against resistance, or he may perform a diagnostic test known as Finkelstein's test. To conduct this test, the doctor will have you flex your thumb into your palm. He will then gently pull the thumb out and down. Wrist pain in response to this test signals possible deQuervain's syndrome.

Tendinitis

This disorder consists of the inflammation of a tendon and adjacent muscle tissue, resulting from the repeated abduction, or pulling away, of a limb from the part of the body to which it's attached. While it's not unusual to develop tendinitis in the wrist, shoulder tendinitis is one of the most common degenerative shoulder diseases seen in industry. In fact tendinitis has been an important cause of missed work and insurance claims for at least sixty years. Wrist tendinitis may develop from jobs that require a lot of twisting motions, such as turning a knob often during the day. Symptoms of tendinitis include pain, swelling, redness, and tenderness of the afflicted part, and sometimes partial loss of function of the fingers or hand.

Tennis Elbow

Also called epicondylitis or lateral epicondylitis, tennis elbow is a painful and sometimes disabling inflammation of the muscles and surrounding tissues of the elbow. It results from repeated strain or inward twisting of the forearm, as might occur not only in tennis but at a job that involves twisting a screwdriver or carrying a heavy load with the arm extended. The main symptoms of tennis elbow are pain and swelling where the tendons and bones meet the elbow joint. A variation of this disorder, called golfer's elbow, results from repeated outward twisting of the forearm, as is commonly done while playing golf.

Raynaud's Syndrome

Repeated exposure to heavy vibration, such as operating a power drill or a chain saw, damages blood vessels in the fingers and may lead to Raynaud's syndrome, also known as Raynaud's phenomenon, vibration white finger disease (VWDF), white finger, or dead finger. The loss of blood flow to the fingers means that less oxygen and nutrients reach the skin and muscle and may lead to the death of that tissue.

Repetitive motion is not always the cause of Raynaud's syndrome. Some people develop an extreme sensitivity to cold temperatures, leading to the shutdown of the blood vessels in their fingers. The causes of this form of the disease, called primary Raynaud's syndrome, or constitutional cold fingers, are still not clear, but many experts believe some people have an inherited tendency for it.

The symptoms of Raynaud's syndrome, primary or job-related, include numbness or tingling in the fingers and hand, loss of heat sensation in that hand, extreme sensitivity to cold, and the possible development of tendonitis or tenosynovitis. Clumsiness and blanching of the skin may also occur, which is why some people call this condition dead finger or white finger disease. Once someone has Raynaud's syndrome, exposure to cold often elicits symptoms.

Some of these symptoms, such as pain, numbness, tingling, and clumsiness, resemble those of CTS, with which Raynaud's syndrome is sometimes confused. That's where some of the above-mentioned diagnostic tests, particularly electromyography, may help make a definite diagnosis. If the affliction is CTS, which is essentially a disorder of the median nerve, nerve-conduction tests should be abnormal. Raynaud's syndrome results from blood vessel damage, so a test of nerve function should yield fairly normal results, although nerve damage is a possibility in very advanced cases. And of course the patient may have Raynaud's syndrome *plus* CTS simultaneously.

Sprains and Strains

People use these terms often and interchangeably, but how many really know what they mean? Doctors think of a *sprain* as an injury to the tendons, or ligaments around a joint, resulting in pain, swelling, and discoloration of the skin over that joint. They define a *strain* as the muscular damage that comes from overzealous physical exertion. The symptoms—pain, redness, heat, and swelling—are similar.

Cysts and Ganglions

Under some circumstances the synovial membrane lining a joint may develop a fluid-filled pouch on or near the joint. The resulting swelling is called a cyst. A ganglion, or ganglion cyst, is a cyst arising from a joint or tendon sheath. Theoretically ganglions may appear anywhere on the body, but they're most commonly found on the wrist or the back of the hand. They usually appear as a smooth, round area of swelling or inflammation and, upon examination, may prove to be attached to the joint or tendon sheath by a stalk. Along with the characteristic swelling and redness, symptoms of a ganglion include pain and possible changes in the size of the mass corresponding with the degree to which the patient uses her hand. No one knows what actually causes ganglions, but many patients have a history of trauma to that wrist, leading some experts to associate it with repetitive motion.

AFTER THE DIAGNOSIS

After reading all of this you may have the impression that accurate diagnosis of an RMD is often a challenge—

and you're right. Once the diagnosis is made, however, treatment is usually straightforward. But that doesn't mean that it's always easy. Sometimes the best way to treat an RMD is to stop the activity that caused it— which isn't realistic if the offending activity is your job! So what can you do? In the chapters that follow, you'll learn more about the treatment of RMDs and the steps you can take if your greatest job hazard does indeed turn out to be the job itself.

THREE

TREATING REPETITIVE MOTION DISORDERS

There's nothing especially mysterious about treating most RMDs, including carpal tunnel syndrome. Soaking in warm water, aspirin, steroids, perhaps a splint or a local anesthetic, and surgery for the more advanced cases form the armamentarium most doctors use to treat these disorders. And in most cases these treatments solve the problem effectively. People may vary in their response to treatment, just as they vary in the pattern and severity of their symptoms, so therapy may work more quickly in one person than in another. Nevertheless the track record for these remedies is good.

The greater challenge lies in preventing RMDs from recurring. You may enjoy a speedy recovery, only to develop the disorder again upon returning to work. That's what happened to Marie, an administrative assistant in a busy real estate firm.

"I had a relatively mild case of carpal tunnel syndrome," she recalls. "The doctor gave me a steroid injection, put my hand in a splint, and told me to rest the hand for a week. Then I went back to work. Everything was fine for about three months or so, and then the pain returned. I stayed on the job as long as I could, but finally the pain got so bad I couldn't move my thumb or my first three fingers anymore. That's when I went back to the doctor, who told me I'd have to have surgery."

The fact is, medical therapy is only half the solution to the problem of RMDs. The other half is changing the nature of your job or working environment—treating the whole workplace, if you will—to prevent the problem from happening again, or ideally, from developing in the first place. This chapter covers the medical treatment of carpal tunnel syndrome and other RMDs; the chapters that follow show the kind of treatment that's available for your job.

TREATING CTS

For mild CTS or symptoms that have persisted for two months or less, most doctors first opt for conservative care: soaking in warm water or wax, warm moist compresses, or wrist immobilization in a splint and the use of painkillers such as aspirin or ibuprofen (because these agents exert a mild anti-inflammatory effect, they're often called nonsteroidal anti-inflammatory drugs, or NSAID). Many people need the splint only at night, while others must wear it around the clock.

Along with the splint and the NSAID your doctor may use steroids to relieve inflammation and pain further. These injections are painless, and their effects may last from a few days to a month or more. CTS should abate as swelling within the carpal tunnel subsides, relieving pressure on the median nerve.

Splints and Steroids

People are sometimes frightened when a doctor decides to use a splint; they associate it with broken bones and other serious injuries. Steroids have developed a bad reputation for dangerous side effects. Yet these two remedies are used frequently in the treatment of carpal tunnel syndrome and many other RMDs, warranting a closer look at each.

Splints. A splint's primary purpose is to immobilize the joint or limb to which it's applied. It makes sense, then, for a doctor to use a splint on a patient with an RMD: The patient may then pursue a relatively normal life while keeping her wrist still. People with tendon disorders of the hand or wrist usually require a splint for three to five weeks.

Splints have other functions as well. Medicine may be applied to the inside surface of the splint, from where it may be absorbed into the skin. In cases where the splint covers an open wound (such as might occur in an accident, but rarely in conjunction with an RMD), it can protect the wound from infection. And by holding the wrist in a stable, comfortable position and keeping it immobilized, a splint may help relieve pain.

It's important to remember that the use of a splint is

not necessarily a reflection of the severity of your case. If anything, the doctor will probably want to use it to prevent your symptoms from becoming *more* severe. Also keep in mind that, by itself, a splint is rarely sufficient to cure an RMD and keep it from returning. That's why it's usually used in conjunction with some other form of treatment, such as steroids.

Steroids.   Not all doctors use steroids in the treatment of CTS, but some believe it is effective. Used to diminish inflammation, the steroids your doctor injects are a version of the steroid hormones produced naturally by your body. These agents act quickly and powerfully to relieve inflammation and its accompanying pain and swelling, which is why they're called anti-inflammatory agents.

Steroids may be given in two forms: orally or by injection. Because they're hormones, steroids may have serious metabolic side effects on many of the body's organ systems. However, these side effects are seen most frequently in people who need high doses of oral steroids for chronic conditions such as arthritis. The small doses you receive by injection for an RMD have a much lower risk of side effects. Besides, if your symptoms don't subside after two or three injections over the course of a few weeks, the chances are you need some other form of treatment, as discussed below. Nevertheless you should be aware of some of the side effects associated with these agents, just to be safe. Such adverse effects include the following: mood swings or personality changes; retention of water or salt; muscle wasting; impaired wound healing; allergic skin reactions; vertigo;

headache; menstrual irregularities; weight gain; excess hair growth; and problems involving the skin around the injection site, including atrophy, lost or excessive pigmentation, and possible abscess formation. If you have cataracts, glaucoma, or a peptic ulcer, warn your doctor before the injection, as steroids may aggravate these conditions.

This list may seem daunting, but remember that most of these effects occur in people who take much higher doses of steroids for a much longer period of time than you'll need for an RMD.

Surgery

If the symptoms resolve after conservative treatment, no other therapy is necessary. Unfortunately these methods are associated with a very high rate of relapse—up to 90 percent, according to some studies—especially if the patient returns to the same job that caused the CTS in the first place. In one experiment patients wore splints for three weeks and received one steroid injection. The researchers then followed their progress for the next eighteen months. The patients with the best outcome had had CTS symptoms for less than one year and normal results on tests of nerve function and muscle mass and strength. The people with the worst outcome were those whose symptoms were more severe and had persisted for more than one year, and whose muscle and nerve function had been impaired, according to diagnostic tests. These patients had the

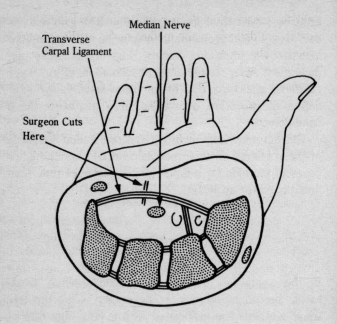

Figure 4. **The transverse carpal ligament is cut during surgery for carpal tunnel syndrome.**

poorest response to therapy and the highest rate of relapse.

If conservative treatment doesn't work, surgery is the next resort. Some doctors use the number of steroid injections a patient needs as a rough guide; the shots should not be administered more than once every two weeks, and if the symptoms return after the third injection, surgery is probably indicated. Surgery is also usually necessary if the doctor determines that there's been extensive damage to the median nerve or the muscles of the thumb.

During surgery for CTS, the doctor simply cuts the transverse carpal ligament, the ligament that runs through the carpal tunnel, as shown in figure 4. This relieves some of the pressure on the median nerve and should allow the symptoms to dissipate. Eventually the ligament heals together again, but it remains wider than it was before, so the operation's therapeutic effects should be intact. The surgeon also removes some of the inflamed synovium that covers the tendon.

To some people the idea of cutting a ligament seems brutal, but in fact this is a fairly routine operation. Most surgeons now do this procedure in the office, with the patient under local anesthesia. The operation lasts thirty to sixty minutes, and the patient can return home that day. In fact many people say they feel better the same evening. To minimize scarring, the doctor usually tries to make the incision in an unobtrusive place, such as the crease of the palm.

Recently some doctors have reported good results with a new technique that is supposed to minimize scarring even further. The surgeon makes a small incision in the palm and the wrist, creating a "tunnel" under the skin. Into this tunnel he inserts an instrument called an endoscope, which is basically a tube with a light attached. He then peers into the tube through a magnifying lens so that he can see the structures of the carpal tunnel and cuts the ligament. The proponents of this method claim that this eliminates the trauma involved with the conventional technique, which requires a larger

FINDING A SURGEON

One way to maximize your chances of a good surgical outcome is to find the best surgeon you can. "The best way to find a good surgeon is to find a happy patient," says one orthopedist, and indeed a referral from a satisfied patient is probably as good a way as any to discover a doctor that's right for you. Ask anyone you know who's had hand surgery recently about her experience and whether she was pleased with her treatment. Alternatively a trusted internist or family physician may be able to put you in touch with a surgeon.

When looking for someone to perform surgery specifically for CTS, it's not enough to find a "hand specialist." Instead you want someone with experience in treating *nerve-entrapment syndromes,* of which CTS is one because it involves swelling and entrapment of the median nerve within the carpal tunnel. This could be a neurosurgeon, an orthopedic surgeon, or even a plastic surgeon who specializes in rehabilitative (as opposed to cosmetic or reconstructive) surgery. The important questions to remember are: how much experience does he have in performing surgery for nerve-entrapment syndromes and how much experience does he have in doing surgery for CTS?

incision so that the entire carpal tunnel may be exposed to view. But other physicians warn that the endoscopic surgery may not permit a good view of the median nerve, leading to the risk of median-nerve damage. Thus while many surgeons agree that the new approach holds promise, more research must be done before it can be used routinely.

Most experts agree that CTS surgery helps virtually every patient who undergoes it. However no one can guarantee that surgery will be 100 percent effective, and it cannot reverse severe nerve or muscle damage—all the more reason to seek help as soon as you notice symptoms. Following the operation, you'll probably have to keep the arm elevated for the next twenty-four hours and try to elevate it as much as possible for the forty-eight hours following that, to minimize swelling. The hand usually remains in a dressing or cast for about two weeks; some doctors make a special splint out of plastic, molded to the patient's hand. It may even be equipped with rubber bands or leather slings to permit rehabilitation exercises. Your hand may feel sore, weak, or numb for up to two months.

Serious or lasting side effects following this operation are rare, but there have been reports of weakened grip, wasting of the muscles at the base of the thumb, persistent pain, loss of finger sensation, and heightened sensitivity to pain in the palm. If you encounter any of these, tell your doctor immediately.

Most doctors prescribe simple exercises to help regain hand and wrist function following surgery; most people can do these on their own, at home. A small percentage of people—one doctor estimates from 10 to 20 percent of his patients—who have greater functional loss may need the services of an occupational therapist, or OT.

Just as many physicians have taken a special interest in disorders of the hand, so have a growing number of OTs. Your specialist may provide exercises designed to restore normal hand and wrist motion, such as squeezing putty, lifting weighted balls, or picking up pegs from a board, and may also have special techniques for relieving pain, such as mild electrical stimulation or immersing the hand in warm paraffin, a method that's described in more detail below.

As you read this, you may be wondering, "What happens after I return to work?" The good news is that surgery should not only cure your CTS, it should prevent it from coming back. But the reality is that there's always a chance CTS or another repetitive motion disorder may recur if you return to the job that caused it. Some experts urge patients to get their companies to redesign the workplace, or even to stop working if necessary. That, of course, is easy for doctors and book writers to say. Most people have no choice but to return to work if they wish to keep paying the rent, or while they hunt for another job. But you're not completely helpless. If you're receiving physical therapy, consider inviting the therapist to your job site, where he or she can watch you work and suggest changes to make your job a little less hard on your hands. Under some circumstances this person may be able to help ease your transition back to work by sending a written report to your boss, your doctor, and your insurance company, stating which tasks you can and cannot do.

Also remember that you now know more about carpal tunnel syndrome—indeed about all the RMDs. Be alert to any abnormal hand sensations and seek help for them promptly.

TREATING THE OTHER RMDS

Along with the remedies used for carpal tunnel syndrome, doctors may rely on two more standbys to treat certain other RMDs. These are ice massage and ultrasound.

Ice Massage

This consists of nothing more than rubbing the inflamed area with an ice cube to reduce pain and swelling.

Ultrasound

Ultrasound involves the transfer of sound waves through the body using a machine designed for that purpose. These sound waves produce heat at the injured site— the tendon or joint capsule—which in turn changes the metabolism in the tissue at that site in a way that promotes healing.

There are two techniques for administering ultrasound therapy. If your injury involves an uneven body surface—a knuckle, perhaps, or a finger joint—or if the area is extremely tender and sensitive to touch, you'll probably receive underwater ultrasound. Your hand will be placed in a water bath, with the sound wave transducer (the component that transmits the sound waves) also in the water bath, about ½ to 1 inch away. Sound waves travel freely through water, so they'll easily reach your hand.

The second method, the direct-contact technique, is often used for acute injuries such as a sprain or strain. Twenty-four to forty-eight hours after the injury occurs, your doctor or therapist will place the sound wave transducer directly on the injured site for about five to eight minutes. The treatments may be administered at least three times a week, and sometimes as often as every day. Most people require about ten sessions in all. If you do have a sprain or strain, it should be treated with ice massage, elevation, and compression with an Ace bandage for the day or two before ultrasound treatments begin.

Now that you're acquainted with the most popular forms of treatment, let's see how they're applied to the different RMDs.

Tenosynovitis.   Most cases of tenosynovitis seem to respond well to a period of immobilization in a splint. Occasional cases may also require a steroid injection.

Advanced cases of tenosynovitis or those affecting certain key joints, such as the thumb, may need more elaborate care. Athletes are particularly prone to developing this form of RMD. Along with splinting and steroids, persistent cases may require a course of therapy with ultrasound or ice massage.

Trigger finger.   For mild cases of trigger finger (those in which the symptoms have occurred for only a few weeks), an injection of steroids directly into the tendon sheath is often all that's needed. Doctors sometimes refer to the "rule of threes" : It may take up to three days for the injection to exert its effects, which then last up to three weeks, and if symptoms return after the third injection, operate.

Surgery for trigger finger involves cutting a portion of damaged tendon sheath through a transverse incision in the finger, restoring free movement to the tendon. Surgery for most RMDs is done quickly and easily, and the patient can return home the same day, just as with surgery for carpal tunnel syndrome.

Some rare cases of trigger finger have been known to resolve on their own, but this isn't something to count on.

DeQuervain's syndrome.   As with CTS, the initial treatment for deQuervain's syndrome consists of splinting, administration of NSAIDs, and possible steroid injections. Some doctors also recommend hot compresses. If these measures don't bring relief within four weeks, surgery is the answer once again. For this disorder, the surgeon will cut the tendon sheath in the portion of the wrist known as the radial aspect, which is the area near the thumb.

Tendinitis.   The treatment for tendinitis is essentially the same as the treatment for tenosynovitis, described above.

Raynaud's syndrome.   Some doctors believe there's no real treatment for Raynaud's syndrome; they contend that the disease may resolve on its own if the patient is young enough and healthy and the offending activity is stopped. But other experts believe there are remedies available to offer at least symptomatic relief. If you have Raynaud's and smoke cigarettes, stop smoking! Your circulation may improve and hence more oxygen and nutrients will be able to reach the tissue damaged by the disease. For those whose pain or discomfort is especially severe, the doctor may prescribe painkillers or inject a local anesthetic into the area.

Sprains and strains.   To treat a sprain or a strain, many experts rely on RICE—rest, ice, compression, and elevation. In other words rest the afflicted area, employ ice massage, compress it by wrapping a bandage around it, and keep it elevated. Ultrasound therapy may also help.

Cysts and ganglions.   The best treatment for these fluid-filled sacs is to let the doctor puncture them in one or more places and allow the fluid to drain out. This is usually followed by an injection of steroids and the application of a special dressing to be worn for forty-eight to seventy-two hours following the puncturing.

Should your symptoms persist despite this treatment, the doctor may decide to remove the cyst surgically. After such a procedure, the chances of recurrence are slim.

As you've seen, treatment for carpal tunnel syndrome and the other RMDs is generally straightforward, even routine for a physician who specializes in hand disorders. Occasionally you may hear of someone who needed multiple operations, or has lots of scars, or experienced lasting damage to her hand, wrist, or arm. Indeed these cases do occur, but these patients are in the minority. So if you've been delaying diagnosis or treatment because you're afraid of dire consequences, rest assured that they are unlikely. As you know, having your symptoms diagnosed *early* and receiving proper care for them is one of the best ways of avoiding serious repercussions.

PREVENTING
WORKPLACE HAZARDS:
THE HUMAN FACTOR

Every day you talk to your television.

Unless of course you don't own a television. Then you probably talk to your car, your radio, your electric blanket, or your elevator. Or your stove, air conditioner, or food processor. Every time you press a button, flip a switch, or turn a dial, you're communicating with the machine to which it's attached. You're telling that machine to change its operation in some way: changing channels on the television, lowering the volume on the radio, adjusting the thermostat in your air conditioner, and so on.

When you work with a machine day in and day out, a control's size, shape, and location on the console are among the factors influencing your comfort and efficiency, not to mention your risk of developing an RMD. In fact virtually every aspect of your workplace, from the level of lighting and the comfort of the furniture, to the way you get along with your boss and co-workers, affects your chances of developing some job-related disorder. A growing number of experts are now turning their attention to the needs of the people who must function in these workplaces every day.

There is a discipline that accounts for human factors in the design of equipment, tools, furniture, and offices. It's been around for many years, and as the current rash of RMDs alerts employers and politicians to the importance of good workplace design, it promises to become more and more important in the years to come. The name of this discipline is ergonomics. In the next few pages you'll learn a little about ergonomics and how its principles can help make for a safer workplace.

ERGONOMICS

The word *ergonomics* combines two Greek words, *ergon* and *nomos,* meaning "work" and "law," respectively. Thus the word itself embodies the concept that work must obey certain laws of human physiology. Some people also refer to this science as human-factors engineering, because it takes human factors into account. *Industrial hygiene* is another term for essentially the same field. People who work in this field are called ergonomists, human-factors engineers, or industrial hygienists.

Ergonomics operates from one basic principle: Make the job fit the person, instead of making the person fit the job. Or as one ergonomics professor explains it,

"Ergonomics concerns the fit between people and the things they use. It's involved with the 'user-friendliness' of objects." While people have suffered job-related injuries for about as long as mankind has been going to work, the increasing complexity of many machines over the past twenty years or so has hastened the development of many RMDs. For example compare the functions of a typewriter to those of a computer workstation. No matter how advanced your typewriter might have been, you still had to keep your files in another location, and you had to use a telephone or intercom to communicate with someone in another office. You also had to stop typing periodically to change paper. VDTs have done away with all that. With these machines, far more complex and versatile than any typewriter, you not only type documents, you can store them on a disk; and many office computer networks allow employees to "talk" to each other via their computer terminals. You rarely have to leave your VDT at all. And that of course is how the seeds of a repetitive motion disorder are sown. Delighted with the prospects of greater productivity, employers introduced VDTs into the workplace with little thought as to how they would change the lives of the people who had to use them.

American engineers first began using ergonomic principles in World War II, when military designers noticed inconsistent control designs between airplanes of different models. They found that a better-designed cockpit increased the pilot's accuracy and stamina. The word *ergonomics* was coined after the war, in 1949. Ergonomic principles were first introduced into the workplace in Europe.

Today ergonomic design affects every facet of life. Human-factors engineering has influenced the design of such consumer items as toys, cars, cameras, and even packages of microwaveable food. This isn't surprising when you realize that ergonomics concerns the interactions between people and objects or machines. It's much easier to change the design of a tool or a computer keyboard than it is to adjust the human body. Even such seemingly minor details such as dials, controls, and instrument panels fall into the realm of ergonomics, along with the design of safety devices, the setup of outside factors such as lighting, and even the organization of the work itself. At first it may seem trivial to worry about something like the design of a control button and the amount of force needed to hit it, but when your job has you pressing that button five thousand times a day—not farfetched if you hit the button once every five seconds or so—poor design becomes a major source of physical stress. In short, ergonomics concerns itself with the design of work equipment, methods, and environments that maximize productivity while minimizing risk.

Human-factors specialists arrive at these designs through a thorough analysis of a job, including the tasks involved, the tools used, and the work environment. They realize that the dimensions of objects in the workplace, such as the height of a desk, chair, or workstation, must match the employee's dimensions—her height, or the length of her arms, for example—as closely as possible. They also know the importance of less tangible factors, such as the number and duration of breaks. Using their knowledge of human anatomical, physiological, and psychological limitations, they apply their findings to develop a workplace that lowers stress and diminishes the risk of disorders such as CTS.

One of the problems still facing ergonomists today is the contrast between the military origins of ergonomics and its current role in the workplace. Military designers were concerned with the efficacy with which soldiers could operate their machinery, and they developed certain design principles based on their experience with physically fit young men. Industrial designers must consider productivity first, and they also must deal with a widely varied work force, many of whose members are not nearly as young and as fit as servicemen. Thus one of the challenges confronting modern ergonomists is to design a workplace that can accommodate people of many different sizes and shapes. Fortunately most of the people in a given work force will fall within certain physical limits—of height, for example, or arm or leg length—and ergonomists can design accordingly. But this means that those people who do fall outside the limits of "average" must either endure more discomfort than most or they must have certain adjustments made for them.

Sometimes the solution to a problem is fairly simple. For example if you've been to an airport recently, you may have noticed that the airline ticket agents had the option of sitting or standing as they worked at their computer terminals. This allows the agents to rest when they want to and to vary their hand positions as they do their job.

Other situations are more complicated. In these cases the expert might break down a job into its component tasks and identify the troublesome ones. For example suppose you work on an assembly line. Your job requires you to assemble one component of an automobile, using parts stored in a bin on a shelf above your head, and then to send that component on down the line. An industrial hygienist might break down your job into the following group of tasks:

- Reach for a part from a storage bin

- Grasp the part

- Move it to the assembly table

- Assemble the item under manufacture

- Release the item along a conveyor belt

Any or all of these motions may require extreme flexion of the wrist (for example the storage bin may have high walls and be located above your head, forcing you to raise your arm and flex your wrist to reach in), pinching with excessive force (as when pulling the part out of the bin), or other actions known to lead to CTS. In addition the scientist may notice that your wrist rubs against the edge of the bin as you remove a part, or that your forearm rubs against the edge of the assembly table as you work. Once the problems are identified, the solutions are often simple: Place the bin below elbow height to prevent excessive flexion of the wrist; dull the bin's sharp edges so that the chances of wrist irritation are reduced; and redesign the assembly table to have sloping edges so that your forearms don't rub against it. It's not unusual for an industrial hygiene specialist to break down a job into twenty component tasks, of which perhaps only two or three are especially stressful. If nothing can be done to ameliorate these tasks, the industrial hygienist may recommend that line employees rotate jobs, perhaps every two hours, so that no one person performs a stressful task too often.

But changes in the workplace aren't always this straightforward. Human-factors engineers sometimes need elaborate tables and charts, detailing exactly what each job in a company entails, the layout of the work area, the tools to be used, and so on. The designer may also have to account for a variety of human factors, such as the workers' height, plus the length of their arms. Computer programs now exist to evaluate stressful tasks, help design new workplaces and work methods, and provide simulations of stress on the body from different work positions, showing the industrial hygienist the least stressful position for any given job. Movies or videotapes of workers in action may also help, for when run in slow motion they enable the expert to spot problems that may previously have gone unnoticed, such as a sudden twisting of the worker's spine or bending of her wrist.

You've read elsewhere in this book that many people don't seek treatment for carpal tunnel syndrome early enough because they don't realize that it might have something to do with their work. Indeed even after reading to this point, you may be hard-pressed to determine whether or not your job puts you at higher-than-average risk of carpal tunnel syndrome or any other RMD. True, we've said that these conditions are associated with awkward, repetitive motions of the arms, wrists, and hands, but what does that really mean? It's hard to pretend you're an industrial hygienist, who can step back and take an objective look at the work you're doing, figure out the various separate tasks involved, and decide if they consist of the sort of activity that might lead to an RMD. What follows, then, is a rundown of some of the jobs most commonly associated with RMDs, and why they seem to cause these problems. You'll also learn some of the criteria you can use to evaluate the risks on your own job and what you can do if your job does make you vulnerable.

HIGH-RISK JOBS: IS YOURS ONE OF THEM?

Here's a partial list of jobs that have been associated with CTS:

Poultry trimming

Fish filleting

Butchering

Meat cutting

Carpet stitching

Sewing and upholstering

Weaving

Garment cutting

Assembly work on a bench

Electronics assembly

Letter sorting

Stone cutting

Riveting

Journalism

Word processing
Piloting a helicopter
Aircraft assembly
Cooking and housecleaning
Playing a musical instrument
Carpentry
Sign language interpretation
Telephone directory assistance
Supermarket checker
Milking cows

If you're starting to think that almost no job is free of risk, you may be right! The fact is, musculoskeletal injuries—those injuries involving the muscles, bones, tendons, ligaments, or joints—are the most common workplace injuries, accounting for 30 to 40 percent of all workers' compensation claims. CTS is one of the most frequently reported of these, along with back problems and sprains and strains.

As you've seen, median-nerve compression caused by swollen tendons in the carpal tunnel is what's responsible for the symptoms of CTS, but there are specific job factors that give rise to this condition. Every job in the list above incorporates at least one of these factors; most involve several. They are the following:

Any repetitive labor of the hands, or twisting or hand-wringing motion of the wrist.   This includes any job that involves cutting, assembling small parts, finishing products like cars or furniture, sewing, or cleaning.

A recent survey of 652 industrial workers, male and female, indicated that repetition of certain movements is perhaps the single greatest risk factor for CTS. But it was the combination of repetition *plus* the use of force, as might be needed to lift heavy objects, tighten difficult screws, or press buttons against a lot of resistance, that was particularly devastating. The survey looked at jobs such as buffing, wax assembly (assembling clusters of wax impressions), automatic machine operation, belt sanding (sanding metal parts using a small wheel), and industrial hanger (transferring parts to and from moving overhead racks). Force combined with repetition increased the risk of CTS by more than fivefold over either factor alone.

There is also some evidence that people who translate sign language are among those at increased risk of CTS. Clearly sign language relies completely on the hands, and an interpreter must keep pace with the person who's speaking, no matter how fast or how long that person talks. Interestingly deaf people who use sign language all the time but don't work as sign language interpreters do not exhibit a higher-than-average incidence of CTS, probably because they have more control over the pace of their signing and can take breaks when they wish.

Heavy use of a VDT. Anyone in a job demanding a lot of time at a VDT risks developing carpal tunnel syndrome or some other RMD. Office workers are certainly among the major users of VDTs, but the list also in-

VDT SYNDROME

9to5, National Association of Working Women, is an organization that helps protect the rights of working women, primarily those who perform office work, such as secretaries and administrative assistants (chapter 6 contains information on contacting 9to5). In conjunction with its sister organization, the Service Employees' International Union (SEIU), 9to5 has published a report entitled, "VDT Syndrome: The Physical and Mental Trauma of VDT Work." This document uses thirty-four case histories to illustrate the problems that may occur from extensive use of VDTs. The cases span age groups, geographic regions, and occupations, testifying to the pervasiveness of these problems among people who use VDTs.

According to the report, VDT syndrome is the general name for the range of health problems that affect VDT users. Along with repetitive motion disorders, these problems include vision problems such as eye fatigue and eye strain; musculoskeletal strain of the back, neck, or shoulder; stress and stress-related disorders such as skin rash; and general symptoms of poor health, which may also be stress-related, such as headaches, nausea, dizziness, and chronic exhaustion.

cludes workers you might not think of, such as journalists, telephone operators, insurance claims processors, travel agents, airline reservation agents, and many, many others. Often these jobs are associated with a rapid work pace, heavy work loads, break times that are sometimes inadequate, and the use of equipment that may force the employee to sit or stand in an uncomfortable position while using a terminal that requires extra force, as well as repetition, when striking the keys. Many industries

The document offers the following suggestions for improving working conditions:

- Seek employee suggestions for improving workstation design

- Use flexible, adjustable equipment that follows ergonomic guidelines

- Include an adequate variety of tasks and breaks in a work day

- Stop the practices of establishing work quotas and programming computers to monitor workers (some industries that require heavy telephone use, such as airline reservations or telephone directory assistance, have computers monitor the number of calls a worker takes or makes, how long she spends on each call, the number of seconds between each call, and how long she spends on breaks for lunch and even going to the bathroom)

- Get adequate, employer-provided medical care for eye and musculoskeletal problems

- Have union contracts insert specific requirements for protecting employees

have started correcting these factors, but some still lag behind.

Tasks that increase pressure in the carpal tunnel. According to a recent study on tasks leading to median-nerve compression, such disparate occupations as milking cows, ladling soup, or even spraying paint from a can, using the index and middle fingers to press the button, all raised carpal tunnel pressure.

Occupations that involve rapid hand motion, that force the worker to assume poor posture while working, or that impose stress on the base of the palm.   Telephone directory assistance jobs, which emphasize answering as many calls as possible during a shift, certainly fall into this category. Jobs that require the use of scrapers, screwdrivers, buffers, or paintbrushes not only involve repeated twisting of the wrist; the tools of these trades also place great stress on the palm. And some people have jobs requiring them to hit the control buttons on machines as rapidly as four to five times a second, adding up to five thousand times a day or more, even allowing for breaks. Hand position and the force needed to get the button pushed are critical in this situation; good equipment design may help the worker stave off CTS.

Use of equipment that vibrates, such as power drills or electric saws, sanders, or buffers.   Gripping the wheel of some kinds of vehicles, such as tractors, may also expose the hands to excessive vibration. Experts still aren't sure why these occupations may lead to CTS, but the jobs and the syndrome have been linked.

Use of machines that have "collars" (safety devices that prevent the accidental activation of a switch).   This equipment is meant to protect the worker, but it may also force him or her to assume an awkward hand position that places stress on wrist tendons.

Frequent reliance on a "pinch" hand position. This is a position that someone might use to grab a narrow board with the fingers, for example. Such a posture demands four to five times more muscle strength and tendon force than a grip position, in which the worker holds the object firmly in his hand, using the palm for support.

Other signals. Some of the other danger signals experts look for include the following:

- Any situation requiring prolonged flexion or extension of the wrist

- Working for long periods with the arms stretched and elbows straight

- Job sites that have controls or materials beyond the comfortable reach of the worker, as in the example just given of the worker who must reach over her head to get a part

- Prolonged operation of heavy or vibrating tools

- Working for long periods with the neck or spine bent, or leaning over frequently

- Excessive twisting or stretching of the back

- Slippery tool handgrips

- Chairs or work surfaces at an awkward height

- Repeated pushing or pulling on loads, especially if they're heavy or if any awkward position is involved

- Standing excessively, or prolonged work in an immobile position

A professional might also seek evidence of unhealthy work practices, including:

- Resting the wrists on the sharp edge of a work surface

- Working on a work surface that's too high, so that the worker has to keep her wrists flexed to get the job done

- Similarly working on a work surface that's tilted away from the worker, so that she has to keep her wrists flexed

These situations may be improved by making sure the work surface is horizontal and at the right height, with padded edges for the arms to rest against without risk of irritating tendons.

EVALUATING YOUR WORKPLACE

When evaluating your job and workplace, it might help to ask yourself the following questions:

1. Do I have enough space to perform my job comfortably?

2. Do I feel tired, weak, or sore while working? If so, where does it hurt? Does it hurt after work or only while I'm on the job? What relieves the pain?

3. Can I think of a better layout for the equipment, storage areas, and work areas I use?

4. How might the equipment and workbench I use better meet my needs? Am I comfortable working with these items, and if not, how might they be changed?

5. Do my tools or work surfaces have any sharp edges? How often do I rub my wrists or arms against those edges?

6. Do I have enough light? How bad is the glare?

7. Are the instruments I need to get the job done— dials, controls, switches, displays, and so on—properly lit, easy to reach, and easy to understand?

8. Does the overall workplace design allow for adequate maintenance and repair?

9. Is there a better way of accomplishing the same task?

WHAT CAN YOU DO ABOUT YOUR WORKPLACE?

Okay, you're in a job that places you at risk of CTS. But what can you do about it?

This chapter opened with a discussion of the science of ergonomics, which helps design jobs and work sites to fit the worker. You can use some of the basic principles ergonomists have developed to help make your job and workplace more worker friendly. Some of these are simple tasks you can try yourself; others may require the cooperation of fellow employees or management. But don't despair if you think you're too far down on the corporate ladder to have any power. You may be able to influence your employer more than you realize. As elected officials become increasingly aware of the problem of RMDs, they're imposing more and more rules protecting workers' rights and health. Infraction of these rules often carries stiff fines, so it's in a company's best interests to listen to the requests of their employees and accommodate them whenever possible.

The rest of this chapter is devoted to steps you and/or your employer can take to provide a safer working environment. Chapter 5 describes your legal options should your employer need a little more persuasion.

Maintain Proper Wrist Position

Stand with your arms hanging relaxed at your side. Note the position of your wrist; it's more or less in a straight line with your hand and forearm. This is the position you should maintain at work, as much as you can. Perhaps you can change the level of your work surface. Some people use books or boards to raise the work surface, while those who must lower it may change to a different work area, cut off or remove the surface's legs, or raise themselves by sitting on one or more pillows, or by standing on books or boards. The important thing is to avoid keeping your wrist bent for long periods of time, especially toward the palm.

Grip

Grip items firmly, so that the object rests in your palm and your fingers' main duty is to keep it from falling (instead of holding the item). Avoid grabbing or "pinching" objects by holding them in your fingers only.

Be Careful How You Use Your Hands After Work

If your job involves high-risk activities, don't compound the risk by spending lots of your leisure time sewing, gardening, playing an instrument, or performing other tasks requiring intensive use of your hands. To the extent that it's possible, avoid sleeping on your hands or lying with the palms bent down.

Create Comfort On the Job

Do as much as you can to create a comfortable working environment. Industries and companies vary in the amount of freedom they give their employees to change working conditions, but if you can, make sure you've got good lighting and ventilation, a comfortable temperature, furniture and equipment that is at least minimally adjustable to your needs, and adequate time for lunch and rest breaks. Use whatever options you have to arrange these factors to your best advantage.

Alert the Company to Uncomfortable Conditions

As mentioned, many employers are more responsive than you might think when told that certain conditions are causing employee discomfort and might possibly lead to the development of RMDs. If your symptoms persist despite your own best efforts, report them to the company doctor or nurse as soon as possible. If you've identified specific elements responsible for the problem—a tool or an uncomfortable piece of furniture that you can't adjust, for example—alert your supervisor or shop steward.

Request Professional Job Analysis

You might suggest to your supervisor that your company consult an ergonomist or industrial hygienist, who can perform time-and-motion studies of specific jobs, and reduce each job to a sequence of motions for each hand. By studying these motions and the frequency with which they're performed, the consultant can pinpoint the factors most likely to cause the development of RMDs and recommend ways of changing them.

Insist Upon Following Government Recommendations

The Occupational Safety and Health Administration (OSHA) has developed three simple suggestions for redesigning jobs and workstations to better fit workers' needs and reduce the risk of injury. They are: use better-designed tools; increase the variety of tasks performed by each worker and decrease the number of repetitions; and provide training in safe work practices. (Note: Chapter 5 discusses the role of OSHA in protecting workers' safety in more detail.)

Encourage Improving Tool Design

A good place to start revamping many tools is at the handle. Changes in handle diameter and length can make the tool easier to grip and relieve some of the force irritating the hand's tendons and nerves. The handle's surface is also important: A napped surface is easier to hold onto than a smooth one and may further reduce stress. In addition some tools come in different sizes or may be adjusted to accommodate the size of the worker's hand. Encourage your employer to provide you with such tools whenever possible. And changes in the angle of certain handles may eliminate the need for awkward wrist postures. Some kinds of pliers, for example, now come with handles bent at a right angle to the working end, so that the worker may keep his hand in a comfortable position while the tool can still reach the work surface.

Sometimes it is possible to minimize the worker's exposure to strong vibration by suspending power tools on balances that support the tool's weight, relieving the hands of considerable weight and force.

Change the Variety of Tasks and the Number of Repetitions

This may be more difficult to accomplish, because it means changing the very nature of the job. It's still possible, however, primarily through the scheduling of more frequent rest breaks, which cuts down on repetition, and having workers rotate among different jobs, which adds to the variety of tasks.

Establish Safer Work Practices

Sometimes a little knowledge is all people need to change their work habits and lower their risk of RMDs or any injury. The National Institute of Occupational Safety and Health (NIOSH) and OSHA both have information on obtaining training for better job safety; in addition people who specialize in ergonomics or industrial hygiene may also be available to train employees. Local hospitals, orthopedics clinics, or college or university departments of physiology may be able to provide information on contacting experts in this field.

Sherry, a supermarket cashier who'd started to notice some aching in her wrists, was skeptical when her store chain invited a local expert in industrial hygiene to speak. "I figured, what could some college professor know about being a grocery checker?" she says now. "But my hands were starting to feel really weak and tired after my shifts, so I figured, the company is giving us this, I have nothing to lose." She was surprised at what she learned. "He explained how we could sit or stand in different positions to decrease the strain in our arms. But the best advice he gave was something so simple, it never occurred to me on my own. He said that probably the best people to learn from were the workers who had been there a long time without any problems, because they'd obviously learned how to get the job done without too much risk to their health." Shaking her head, she adds, "Doesn't that seem obvious? If you want to find something out, ask the person who's been on the job the longest. But I would never have thought of it if he hadn't mentioned it."

ENLIGHTENED SELF-INTEREST

There are still some businesses that, for a variety of reasons, hesitate to make the changes that would lower their employees' risk of RMDs or other occupational disorders. That's why, when all else fails, you can resort to the legal actions described in chapter 5. Fortunately, however, more and more employers are learning that it's in their best interest to provide their workers with a safe and comfortable workplace. In the words of one distinguished ergonomist:

"Perhaps the ergonomist should approach a potential employer not with any claim to improving productivity but rather to improve safety and reliability and to maintain the long-term health of the employees. The employer should invest in ergonomics not to increase his profits but because it is his inescapable responsibility to his employees." *

* Singleton, W.T., ed. *The Body at Work: Biological Ergonomics.* Cambridge, Eng.: Cambridge University Press, 1982.

LEGAL MANEUVERS

When should an employee take legal action against her employer? Is she better advised to fight for changes through whatever company-sanctioned channels exist? Or should she continue to suffer in silence, perhaps while hunting for a new job?

All of these options have risks. Lawsuits can take years and bring no end of stress and aggravation. What's worse, the worker may be branded a "troublemaker" by her company—indeed, perhaps by an entire industry— and may never be able to find a job in that field again. And there's always the risk of losing the suit, which means the plaintiff will have gained nothing and may be left with a mountain of lawyers' bills. Clearly this is a measure of last resort.

Working for change through official channels may be preferable, providing the company *has* channels for employees to get their grievances heard and acted upon when appropriate. Here again, however, the employee who presses her case too vigorously risks developing a reputation as a troublemaker, which could affect her opportunities for raises or promotions.

Finally there's always the option of simply staying on the job and quietly searching for new employment. But once more, there are problems. It may take months, indeed possibly a year or even more, to find a new job. If someone is already experiencing symptoms of an RMD, she may do herself irreparable harm by continuing to perform the same work. Indeed she may get to the point where she may be unable to work at all. And if she finds a job doing the same kind of work, she'll be in the same situation, unless her new employer offers better working conditions.

The ideal situation, then, would appear to be one in which an employer allows workers to report health risks as they perceive them and is willing to make changes based upon the recommendations of employees and perhaps professional ergonomists. Of course if you are represented by a union, you can also turn to your local for help.

HOW A UNION MAY HELP

Employees in many industries have unions to represent them in grievances and negotiations with management. The guidelines for bringing a grievance vary according to the union and its agreements with the company. Basically, however, you must first have your disorder documented by a physician—your own or one designated by your employer or an insurance company. If, however, you don't obtain relief after thirty days' treatment by a doctor chosen by someone else, you then have the right to have your case confirmed by a physician of your own choosing.

Once it's been established that the disorder is work-related (not always easy when the disorder is an RMD), you should first talk to someone at your company about your options—obtaining medical care, workers' compensation, extra sick time, changes in your work environment, and so on. Here again, there are no set rules; the procedure varies from business to business. In a small company where things are informal, you may be able to go straight to the president. In large corporations with hundreds of employees, you'd most likely see someone in the personnel or human resources department. In any case if you're a union member, you should notify the appropriate official—shop steward, union representative, committeeman; here, too, it varies with the union.

The union acts officially if you don't receive satisfaction from your employer. It can investigate the situation, see if other workers are suffering from the same problem, and negotiate with management for a settlement that's acceptable to all parties (although state or federal regulations dictate the ultimate limits of the settlement—the union settlement must be within these guidelines). Your union can also put you in touch with an attorney who can help you pursue a workers' compensation claim, should that be necessary. And if your union is large and powerful enough, if a large number of workers are affected, and if the problem is particularly egregious, it can help its members sue a business into making changes.

EXAMPLE:
THE CASE AGAINST US WEST

The Communications Workers of America (CWA), the union that represents telephone operators, recently filed suit against US West, a Denver telephone company, due to a rash of RMDs among its employees there. Between 1986 and 1989, 189 US West operators—about one-third of the work force—reported such disorders. Of these, about seventy, or roughly one of every seven employees, developed carpal tunnel syndrome. Ten of these workers were fired because management felt they could no longer keep up with the demands of the job.

Telephone operators are among the heaviest users of VDTs: As requests for phone numbers come in, the operators call up the information from the VDT. An average operator at US West answered up to twelve hundred calls per day, or one call every twenty-four seconds. The computer recorded this information and printed it out daily. Each operator had a quota of calls to take. The rapid work pace and constant pressure to perform, added to the poorly designed VDT stations, placed these workers at particularly high risk of repetitive motion disorders.

Recognizing the risks of heavy VDT use since the early 1980s, CWA had negotiated with several telephone companies for VDT workplace design guidelines. But the growing incidence of RMDs among their workers (including thousands who worked for companies other than US West) convinced the union that management had not been making the agreed-upon improvements.

The US West suit arose out of frustration that management did not seem to take the workers' needs seriously—instead it laid off workers who became disabled when they were simply trying to do their job. To be fair, US West executives later admitted that when the first few reports of RMDs began trickling in, the company, unfamiliar with these conditions, didn't believe the disorders had anything to do with work. Management became more sympathetic as the trickle became an avalanche.

Nevertheless the union turned to the Occupational Safety and Health Administration (OSHA), the federal agency charged with protecting workers' rights to a safe and healthy workplace. OSHA reviewed the case and cited the company for serious violations. The agency noted that operators could not adjust the position of their VDT screens, keyboards, and chairs. It also found that the keys were difficult to press. The charges were dropped only after US West agreed to replace the equipment and teach operators about injury prevention.

In all, US West spent some $2 million to redesign its offices and equipment, and more than another $2 million on the medical care of the afflicted workers. Lawyers and outside consultants cost the company at least $1 million more, bringing the total to over $5 million. US West might have been able to save as much as $3 million of that had it made the workplace changes when they were first requested.

BUILDING A CASE

What if you don't belong to a union that can look after your interests? Don't despair—there are steps "little people" can take on their own.

First of all, gather evidence to support your suspicions. If you've got what you think are symptoms of CTS or a related disorder, chances are others in your company do, too, more evidence that these conditions are associated with occupation.

"I knew my symptoms were work-related when I started talking to some of the other secretaries in my office and to friends I had who worked in other companies that used the same equipment," says Randi, a legal secretary with fifteen years' experience. "About three years ago my law firm got a new computer system with new word-processing software. My hands started aching and tingling, first at night, sometimes bad enough to wake me up. At first I didn't relate it to work, so I'm not sure exactly when it started, but I would guess it began about six months after we got the new equipment. Then my hands started to ache all the time. I went on vacation a few months later, and after about a week away from the job, I noticed my hands were feeling better. They got worse again when I returned to work. That's when I realized that the aches and pains were job-related." Randi's employer was enlightened enough to give her plenty of time off for doctor visits and therapy, but not enough to consider revamping the computer system. Her symptoms returned as soon as she went back to her job. "That proved to me beyond any doubt that the problem was with that computer," she recalls. "What made it even scarier was that some of the other secretaries were also starting to develop symptoms."

You can start building your case by doing what Randi did: Seek a pattern to any symptoms you might have. Do your hands feel better after a vacation or a long weekend? Do your symptoms return when you go back to work? Can you associate your condition with any job changes that have occurred within the last six to twelve months? (This includes not just starting a new job but any changes in procedure or equipment that have occurred on a current job.) Keep a diary of your symptoms, recording what they are, when they occur, and when they subside. Written documentation is invaluable during legal negotiations.

Company records are also significant. You can identify jobs with a high risk of RMDs by examining employee health data, such as logs of medical visits or first-aid administration, reports from a worker's own doctor, workers' compensation data, and the logs that OSHA requires many industries to keep. Not all employees have access to this information, but if you do, study it.

As Randi discovered, co-workers may also be valuable sources of information. Keep abreast of company gossip; learn who's out sick and why. Does your workplace have a high incidence of sprains, strains, or tendonitis? These disorders often result from the same conditions that produce carpal tunnel syndrome and other RMDs, and sometimes they presage their development.

Once you've accumulated evidence of a problem, you can get government assistance by following these steps:

1. Call the National Institute of Occupational Safety and Health (NIOSH), in Cincinnati, Ohio, at (513) 841-4382.

2. Ask to speak to someone in the Hazard Evaluation Technical Assistance branch.

3. The official, or project officer, who speaks to you will be able to answer questions, provide information, and help you get a better perspective on your situation. Should you wish to have NIOSH review your case and possibly inspect your workplace, ask the official to send you a Health Hazard Evaluation (HHE) form (see Figure 5 on page 95.)

4. Complete the HHE form. NIOSH has estimated this step to take about twelve minutes. You'll be asked to provide the signatures of two other employees who also believe there's a problem. *This information is held strictly confidential at your request. Your employer need never know who asked for the evaluation.* A copy of the HHE form is shown on pages 95–97.

5. Send the form back to NIOSH. The agency will review it and have a project officer contact you. Based on the information you provide, NIOSH may make some recommendations to you or your employer, or it may send the project officer to your workplace for a firsthand evaluation. NIOSH's aid is free to employee and employer. Even if the employer is found to be in violation, a penalty may not be levied if the company seems to be acting in good faith and is willing to make the recommended changes.

GOVERNMENT ACTION

Sometimes cases arise in which the federal government must force a recalcitrant employer to adhere to the rules and regulations that assure each worker the right to a safe and comfortable workplace. Companies in certain industries must maintain logs of occupational injuries and periodically submit these to the Occupational Safety and Health Administration—OSHA—for its review. The agency uses this information to concentrate on high-risk industries in general, verifying these reports with other records of illnesses and injury such as company first-aid files, workers' compensation claims, and the medical records of individual employees. When a discrepancy arises between company reports and OSHA information, OSHA inspects the company.

These inspections include reviews of company records as well as of the workplace itself. If OSHA finds safety violations, records of frequent injuries, or other problems, it may issue a citation to that employer. It's then up to the company to evaluate its conditions and develop a detailed plan for rectifying those conditions, including special training sessions for employees, managers, and the medical staff. The training sessions and other improvements must follow a schedule also developed by the company.

Sometimes an OSHA inspector may discover problems that need solutions but aren't serious enough to warrant a citation. In such cases OSHA sends a letter to the company, describing the problem and suggesting ways it can be solved. If the problems still exist in a later inspection, OSHA then cites the company.

Usually an OSHA inspection or citation is enough to make a company improve working conditions. Occasionally, however, the agency encounters violations that are particularly serious, willful, or persistent. In these cases the administration may impose a separate fine for each instance of the particular violation it finds. This can lead to very high penalties for the responsible company, sometimes amounting to millions of dollars.

For example, in July 1987 an OSHA inspection of the Iowa Beef Processing (IBP) plant in Dakota City, Nebraska, revealed 620 willful violations associated with a high rate of repetitive motion disorders, especially carpal tunnel syndrome. Initially OSHA imposed penalties of $3.1 million for the ergonomic violations, plus another $2.6 million for the willful underreporting of illnesses and injuries. IBP finally settled the case for a fine of $975,000, plus agreements to begin a company-wide ergonomics program and to report illnesses and injuries according to federal regulations.

THE PRICE OF GOOD JOB DESIGN

Some companies have used cost as a reason for delaying workplace changes. It's now become clear, however, that the costs of workers' compensation claims, lost work time, other medical expenses, and possible OSHA fines usually equal or exceed the expense of revamping the job. For example remember that US West spent

OSHA AND NIOSH: WHO DOES WHAT?

These two federal agencies work closely together, which isn't surprising since each one's reason for being is, ultimately, to make American workers safer. Beyond that the differences between the two agencies' duties and jurisdictions are sometimes rather fuzzy.

Both agencies were established in the early 1970s, when Congress passed the Occupational Safety and Health Act. OSHA became part of the Department of Labor and was mandated to develop and enforce health standards in the workplace. In its role as a policing agency, OSHA is able to inspect workplaces and levy fines if necessary. Chapter 6 has more information about OSHA.

NIOSH supplies OSHA with much of the information it needs to set workplace health standards. Part of what is today called the Department of Health and Human Services (when NIOSH was first established, the umbrella agency was known as the department of Health, Education, and Welfare), NIOSH's primary job is to research and recommend safety standards for OSHA to set. When the agency performs a health hazard evaluation (HHE), as described above, it sends copies of its records to OSHA for its files. NIOSH also functions as an educational agency, funding university research and teaching projects on occupational safety and health.

about $2 million on new equipment, but by the time it purchased that equipment, lost wages, health care benefits, and legal fees had cost it as much as $3 million more. And while IBP succeeded in lowering its penalties, it still paid nearly $1 million in fines above and beyond the cost of making workplace reforms.

WHO WILL DEVELOP CTS?

Some people have suggested that one way to lower the rate of CTS in the workplace is to screen out any potential employee who may be at higher-than-average risk for the syndrome. Unfortunately there does not yet exist any reliable way to determine who's going to develop CTS in the future. Some studies have suggested that people with small carpal tunnels experience higher rates of CTS, but experts dispute these findings, and most physicians emphasize that, right now, there is no way to screen anyone for CTS—not to mention the possible civil rights questions such a process would raise. It's much easier, and more cost-effective, to make the necessary changes in the design of job, tools, and workplace than it is to try to guess who will someday develop CTS.

HELPING YOURSELF

The goal of this book has been to give you the information you need to take control of your well-being. You have options at every step of the way—from remembering to rest your hands every so often at the first slight signs of an RMD to taking legal action against a stubborn employer. You've learned how you can protect yourself by recognizing the symptoms of carpal tunnel syndrome and other RMDs, seeking effective care and making the appropriate changes in your life and work. The rest is up to you.

Figure 5. Health Hazard Evaluation Form.

Form Approved
OMB No. 0920-0102
Exp. Date Aug. 31, 1992

U.S. DEPARTMENT OF HEALTH AND HUMAN SERVICES
CENTERS FOR DISEASE CONTROL
NATIONAL INSTITUTE FOR OCCUPATIONAL SAFETY AND HEALTH

REQUEST FOR HEALTH HAZARD EVALUATION

This form is provided to assist in registering a request for a health hazard evaluation with the U.S. Department of Health and Human Services. Public reporting burden for this collection of information is estimated to average 12 minutes per response. Send comments regarding this burden estimate or any other aspect of this collection of information, including suggestions for reducing this burden to PHS Reports Clearance Officer; ATTN: PRA, Hubert H. Humphrey Bg, Rm 721-H; 200 Independence Ave., SW: Washington, DC 20201, and to the Office of Management and Budget; Paperwork Reduction Project (0920-0102); Washington, DC 20503. (See Statement of Authority on Reverse Side)

Establishment Where Possible Hazard Exists _____
Company   Street_____Telephone_____
Address
          City_____State_____Zip Code_____

1. Specify the particular building or worksite where the possible hazard/problem is located.

2. Specify the name, title, and phone number of the employer's agent(s) in charge.

3. What Product or Service does the Establishment Produce?

4. Describe briefly the possible hazard/problem which exists by completing the following:

   Identification of Hazardous Physical Agent(s)_____

Identification of Toxic Substance(s)_____

Trade Name(s) (If Applicable)_____Chemical Name(s)_____
_____
_____

Manufacturer(s)_____
Physical Form of Substance(s):_____Dust_____Gas
_____Liquid_____Mist_____Other
How are you exposed? _____Breathing _____Swallowing
_____Skin Contact
Number of People Exposed _____
Length of Exposure (Hours/Day)_____
Occupations of Exposed Employees_____
_____

5. Using the space below describe further the circumstances which
   prompted this request. _____
   _____
   _____

6. To your knowledge has NIOSH, OSHA or any other government
   agency previously evaluated this workplace? _____yes
   _____no

7. (a) Is a similar request currently being filed with or under
       investigation by any other Government (State or Federal)
       agency? _____
   (b) If so, give the name and address of each. _____

   8. Requester's Signature_____Date_____
      Typed or Printed Name_____Phone: Home-_____
             Street_____Business-_____
      Address
             City_____State_____Zip Code_____

9. Check only One of the Following:
   _____ I am an Employer Representative
   _____ I am an Authorized Representative of, or an officer of the
          organization representing the employees for purposes of
          collective bargaining. State the name and address of your
          organization. _____
   _____ I am a current employee of the employer and an
          Authorized Representative of two or more current
          employees in the workplace where the substance is

normally found. Signatures of authorizing employees are below:

Name_____ Phone_____

Name_____ Phone_____

_____ I am one of three or less employees in the workplace where the substance is normally found.

10. Please indicate your desire: _____ I do not want my name revealed to the employer.

_____ My name may be revealed to the employer.

Authority:

Sections 20(a)(3-6) of the Occupational Safety and Health Act, (29 U.S.C. 669(a)(6)) and Section 501(a)(11) of the Federal Mine Safety and Health Act, (30 U.S.C. 951(a)(11)). Confidentiality of the respondent requester will be maintained in accordance with the provisions of the Privacy Act (5 U.S.C. 552a). The voluntary cooperation of the respondent requester is necessary to conduct the Health Hazard Evaluation.

For Further Information:
Telephone: AC 513/841-4382
Send the completed form to:
National Institute for Occupational Safety and Health
Hazard Evaluations and Technical Assistance Branch
4676 Columbia Parkway, Mail Stop R-9
Cincinnati, Ohio 45226

SIX

WHERE TO GO FOR MORE INFORMATION

Want to learn more about CTS or related disorders, how to find a doctor, or what your rights are as an employee? Many organizations, some private, some government-run, exist to help you in your quest.

UNIONS

In an effort to protect their constituents, many unions maintain records of workplace injuries and have gathered information about workers' rights. What follows is a partial list; if one of these organizations cannot answer your questions, they may be able to direct you to someone who can.

International Union of the United Automobile, Aerospace, and Agricultural Implement Workers of America, UAW
UAW Health and Safety Department
8000 East Jefferson
Detroit, Michigan 48214
(313) 926-5566

The UAW represents thousands of workers whose jobs have placed them at risk of most of the conditions discussed in this book. It has several publications on these problems and may be able to refer questioners to sources of help in their own communities.

9to5, National Association of Working Women
614 Superior Avenue, NW
Cleveland, Ohio 44113
(216) 566-9308

9to5 is committed to helping working women gain power on the job in the form of better working conditions, respect from others, and improved self-esteem. The organization offers advice on workers' rights, counseling, and publishes a variety of newsletters and pamphlets on subjects of interest to female workers.

The Newspaper Guild
8611 Second Avenue
Silver Spring, Maryland 20910
(301) 585-2990

The Newspaper Guild represents some forty thousand news industry employees, such as reporters, in the United States, Canada, and Puerto Rico. It has records of hundreds of cases of RMDs that have occurred among employees at newspapers around the country and has documented cases that have occurred in other parts of the world, particularly Australia. Like secretaries and other administrative workers, journalists rely heavily upon VDTs, so perhaps it's not surprising that so many of these workers have contracted some form of RMD. If you spend many hours writing at a computer, you may wish to contact the Newspaper Guild for more information.

GOVERNMENT AGENCIES

The next time you wonder where all your tax money goes, you might want to read about the following organizations. At little or no cost, they will send literature, answer questions, and serve as an all-purpose resource for information about occupational safety and health. Since these are, after all, government agencies, you may have to make more than one call and speak to more than one person to get the information you seek, but rest assured, if it's there, they'll help you find it.

Clearinghouse for Occupational Safety and Health Information
Department of Health and Human Services
Centers for Disease Control
National Institute for Occupational Safety and Health
4676 Columbia Parkway
Cincinnati, Ohio 45226
(513) 533-8385

Established in 1976, the clearinghouse provides information to the public and offers technical support for research programs. The clearinghouse maintains a library containing about twelve thousand books and eleven hundred periodicals and also has a computer data base that indexes information on occupational safety and health going back to the nineteenth century.

Office of Information
National Institute for Occupational Safety and Health
  (NIOSH)
Department of Health and Human Services
Centers for Disease Control
Building 1, Room 3041
1600 Clifton Road, NE
Atlanta, Georgia 30333
(404) 329-3345

This is the office to call if you're a nonscientist with questions about occupational safety and health. Along with information about RMDs, this office also maintains a computer data base on toxic substances in the workplace.

Occupational Safety and Health Administration
  (OSHA)
Office of Information and Consumer Affairs
Department of Labor
200 Constitution Avenue, NW
Room N-3637
Washington, D.C. 20210
(202) 523-8148

OSHA was created in 1970 to encourage employers and employees alike to reduce workplace hazards and to improve safety and health programs or establish ones where none had existed previously. OSHA's mandate also includes the establishment of interdependent rights and responsibilities for workers and managers; to monitor on-the-job injuries and illnesses through proper reporting and record-keeping systems; to develop mandatory job safety and health standards and to enforce them; and to provide for the development, analysis, evaluation, and approval of state occupational safety and health programs. OSHA encourages a broad range of voluntary effort to improve the workplace, such as consultation programs, training and education, grants to increase safety compliance, and other, similar programs.

Along with all of this, OSHA has publications on occupational health and safety, asbestos, hearing, back injuries, accidents, federal regulations, statistical data, and carcinogens. To obtain OSHA publications, contact:

The National Technical Information Service
Port Royal Road
Springfield, Virginia 22161
(703) 487-4650

or:

Superintendent of Documents
U.S. Government Printing Office
Washington, D.C. 20402
(202) 566-2000

FINDING A DOCTOR

Most medical specialties have professional societies that offer help in finding a doctor in local communities. Often they also provide additional resources, such as publications on health issues or certain medical problems. If the information you wish is of a medically related nature, or if you're looking for a physician near you who treats CTS, you might consider calling one of the following organizations.

American Academy of Orthopedic Surgeons
222 South Prospect Avenue
Park Ridge, Illinois 60068-4058
(708) 823-7186

American Medical Association
535 North Dearborn Street
Chicago, Illinois 60610
(312) 645-5000

American Academy of Neurological Surgeons
Department of Neurology
University of Tennessee
956 Court Avenue
Memphis, Tennessee 38163
(901) 528-6374

American Board of Surgery
1617 John F. Kennedy Boulevard
Philadelphia, Pennsylvania 19103
(215) 568-4000

American Society of Plastic and Reconstructive
  Surgeons
444 East Algonquin Road
Arlington Heights, Illinois 60005
(312) 806-9696

American College of Sports Medicine
P.O. Box 1440
1 Virginia Avenue
Indianapolis, Indiana 46206
(317) 637-9200

FOR MORE ON ERGONOMICS

If you're interested in learning more about ergonomics, contact:

The Human Factors Society
P.O. Box 1369
Santa Monica, California 90406
(213) 394-1811

This is a professional society for people who do research on ergonomics.

GLOSSARY

abduction: the act of pulling a limb away from the body.

abductor pollicis brevis: the muscle extending from the base of the thumb to the small bones of the hand. The abductor pollicis brevis bends the thumb and pulls it away from the other fingers; its function may be affected in carpal tunnel syndrome.

acromegaly: a condition resulting from the excessive secretion of pituitary growth hormone. Acromegaly is characterized by distortion of the bones of the face, skull, and feet, as well as the hand, and is occasionally the cause of CTS.

arthritis: a general term for any inflammation of a joint. There are many different forms of arthritis, such as osteoarthritis, rheumatoid arthritis, and gout, to name only three.

arthrogram: an X ray of a joint, using a special dye or contrast medium.

arthroscope: a tube with a light at one end that a physician inserts directly into a joint for a close look at the joint's condition. An arthroscope is one of a group of instruments known as endoscopes, all of which are tubes with lights at one end, specially designed for looking into body cavities.

atrophy: the withering of an organ, such as a muscle.

bilateral: a condition that occurs on both sides of the body. Carpal tunnel syndrome that occurs in both hands is described as bilateral CTS.

biomechanics: the application of the laws of mechanics to living structures.

bursa: a fluid-filled sac situated in areas of the body in which friction would otherwise develop, such as a joint.

bursitis: inflammation of a bursa.

carpal tunnel: the narrow, bony tunnel at the junction of the hand and wrist through which pass the median nerve and nine important tendons.

carpal tunnel syndrome (CTS): the syndrome that results when the tendons in the carpal tunnel become irritated and swollen and press on the median nerve. Symptoms of CTS include pain, numbness, and tingling in the fingers and palm; clumsiness; and loss of grip strength. Advanced cases of CTS may lead to wasting of certain muscles in the hand.

computerized axial tomography (CAT): the use of a computer and specialized equipment to obtain X rays of specific portions of the body; also called CAT scan, computed tomography, or CT scan.

constitutional cold fingers (primary Raynaud's syndrome): see Raynaud's syndrome.

crepitus: a clicking or cracking noise sometimes made by a joint.

cumulative trauma disorder (CTD): a muscle, nerve, or joint disorder caused by the repetition of stressful or awkward movements, usually as part of one's job. Also called repetitive motion injury, repetitive strain injury, or repetitive motion disorder (RMD).

cyst: any closed cavity, normal or abnormal, that contains a liquid or semisolid material.

dead finger: see Raynaud's syndrome.

deQuervain's disease (deQuervaine's disease, deQuervaine's syndrome): a form of tenosynovitis characterized by swelling and inflammation of the tendons going to the base and back of the thumb.

dorsal side: the back side of a body part or organ. The dorsal side of the hand would be the side opposite the palm.

electrode: a conductor that establishes contact with a nonmetallic part (that is, a part that does not normally conduct electricity) to complete an electrical circuit. In medical use electrodes are attached to certain parts of the body to measure the electricity generated by that part of the body. Doctors sometimes use electrodes to help measure nerve or muscle activity when testing for carpal tunnel syndrome.

electromyography (EMG): the science of detecting and analyzing the electrical signals that emanate from muscles in order to evaluate the function of those muscles. EMG is sometimes used in the diagnosis of CTS or other cumulative trauma disorders. (Also see electrode, above).

epicondylitis: pain and swelling of the muscle and tendon surrounding the elbow joint. One of the cumulative trauma disorders, epicondylitis is also known as tennis elbow.

ergonomics: the science of designing tools, offices, and other areas of the workplace to best fit the needs and the physiology of the worker.

extension: stretching or straightening of a joint.

extensor: a muscle that extends a joint.

Finkelstein's test: a diagnostic test for carpal tunnel syndrome in which the doctor gently pulls your flexed thumb out and down. Wrist pain in response to this test signals possible deQuervain's syndrome.

flexion: bending of a joint.

flexor: a muscle that bends or flexes a joint.

flexor retinaculum: a heavy, fibrous band of tissue that composes one of the walls of the carpal tunnel. Also called the transverse carpal ligament.

ganglion: an abnormal cyst that appears near a joint, usually the wrist.

gout: a form of arthritis or joint inflammation caused by the buildup of uric acid in the blood. Gout attacks occur most commonly in the big toe, but in rare cases the wrist may be the site of inflammation.

human factors engineering: see ergonomics.

industrial hygiene: see ergonomics.

ligament: a shiny, white band of flexible tissue that connects the two bones of a joint.

median nerve: the nerve that runs through the carpal tunnel to serve the thumb and the first three fingers of the hand. Pressure on the median nerve from swollen tendons in the carpal tunnel leads to the symptoms of carpal tunnel syndrome.

myxedema: the condition that results from having an underactive thyroid. Myxedema is characterized by a swelling of the skin and abnormal deposits of a material called mucin (a component of mucous) in the skin and other tissues.

palmar: an adjective for something that pertains to the palm of the hand.

Phalen's sign: see Phalen's test, below.

Phalen's test: one of the diagnostic tests for carpal tunnel syndrome, involving extreme flexion of the wrist in question for up to one minute. If symptoms appear within that time period, the likely diagnosis is CTS.

Raynaud's phenomenon: see Raynaud's syndrome, below.

Raynaud's syndrome: a syndrome characterized by numbness or tingling in the hand, loss of heat sensation in the hand, extreme sensitivity to cold, also in that hand, tendonitis, and tenosynovitis. Raynaud's syndrome may be caused by persistent exposure to heavy vibration or extreme cold, but some people develop it for reasons doctors have yet to identify. Also called Raynaud's phenomenon, white finger, dead finger, constitutional cold fingers, or vibration white finger disease (VWFD).

repetitive motion disorder (RMD): a musculoskeletal disorder caused by performing the same awkward motion over and over again. See also cumulative trauma disorder.

repetitive strain injury (RSI): see cumulative trauma disorder and repetitive motion disorder.

sprain: an injury to the tendons or ligaments around a joint, resulting in pain, swelling, and discoloration of the skin over that joint.

strain: muscular damage resulting from overexertion.

synovial joint: a joint whose bony surfaces are covered by cartilage and connected by ligaments lined by a synovial membrane.

synovial membrane: the membrane that lines a synovial joint and secretes a fluid into the joint, helping to keep it lubricated.

synovial sheath (also called synovial tendon sheath): a membranous sac enclosing a tendon that runs through one of the tunnels in the body, such as the carpal tunnel. The sheath secretes a fluid that helps lubricate the tendon, enabling it to glide through the tunnel more smoothly.

synovitis: see tenosynovitis, below.

tendinitis: inflammation of a tendon and some of the adjacent muscle tissue, resulting from the repeated pulling away of the limb from the part of the body to which it's attached. Also called tendonitis.

tendon: a fibrous portion of a muscle that connects it to a bone.

tendonitis: See tendinitis, above.

tennis elbow: see epicondylitis.

tenosynovitis: inflammation of a tendon and the associated synovial sheath, often caused by extreme flexion of the joint. Carpal tunnel syndrome is one form of tenosynovitis. Also called synovitis.

thenar eminence: the fleshy mound at the base of the thumb.

Tinel's sign: tingling or pain in one or more fingers in response to gentle tapping or stroking on the wrist in someone who has carpal tunnel syndrome. Tinel's sign is sometimes used as a diagnostic test for CTS, but a large segment of people with the syndrome do not display Tinel's sign.

torque: a force that produces or tends to produce rotation.

transverse carpal ligament: see flexor retinaculum.

trauma: a general word for injury, but usually implying an injury caused by an accident, crime, or other traumatic event.

trigger finger: a form of tenosynovitis that occurs from excessive flexion of a finger (thumb excluded), particularly against resistance, as when pulling a trigger.

ulnar: the side of the hand opposite the thumb. The term comes from the ulna bone, which is the inner and larger bone in the forearm.

vibration white finger disease (VWFD): see Raynaud's syndrome.

vibrometer: an instrument that measures vibration perception in selected parts of the body, such as the hand.

volar: an adjective for something that pertains to the palm of the hand or the sole of the foot.

white finger: see Raynaud's syndrome.

INDEX

ABOUT THE AUTHOR

Norra Tannenhaus holds degrees in biopsychology and nutrition from Vassar College and Columbia University. She has written extensively on health, medicine, and nutrition for consumers and physicians, and her magazine articles have appeared in such major publications as *Self*, *Glamour*, and *Mademoiselle*. Although she is a New Yorker at heart, Ms. Tannenhaus currently makes her home in Los Angeles. *Relief from Carpal Tunnel Syndrome and Other Repetitive Motion Disorders* is her fifth book. She is also the author of *Learning to Live with Chronic IBS* in the Dell Medical Library.